SHIFT
for GOOD

ALSO BY TORY JOHNSON

The Shift:
How I Finally Lost Weight and Discovered a Happier Life

Fired to Hired:
Bouncing Back from Job Loss to Get to Work Right Now

Spark & Hustle:
Launch and Grow Your Small Business Now

SHIFT
for GOOD

How I Figured It Out and Feel Better Than Ever

TORY JOHNSON

**Waterford City and County
Libraries**

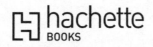
hachette
BOOKS

NEW YORK BOSTON

Hachette Books
Hachette Book Group
1290 Avenue of the Americas
New York, NY 10104
www.HachetteBookGroup.com

Printed in the United States of America

LSC-C

First trade paperback edition: December 2016

10 9 8 7 6 5 4 3 2 1

Hachette Books is a division of Hachette Book Group, Inc.

The publisher is not responsible for websites (or their content) that are not owned by the publisher.

LCCN: 2015023593

ISBN 978-0-316-26158-6 (trade pbk.)

For my mom, who always finds something to celebrate, and to every woman who does her best to make today better than yesterday

Contents

LIFE KEEPS HAPPENING

A NEWER ME

LOVE AND SERVICE

SHIFTING FOR GOOD

Preface

had battled obesity since childhood, a secret shame that haunted me.

As a regular on *Good Morning America*, my biggest fear was being called out about my weight. So three years ago, when my ABC News boss said she didn't think I looked my best and wanted me to see a stylist, what I heard was *lose weight—or lose your job*. Those words never crossed her lips, but that's the message I got loud and clear. Although it was brief, I couldn't wait for our little chat to end. When it was up, I managed to dash from the ABC cafeteria before bursting into tears.

After a good cry at home, I had an honest conversation with myself about my forty-year battle of the bulge. *Enough is enough*, I thought. *It's time to lose weight once and for all. No more gimmicks. No more lies. No more excuses. You're a smart girl. Figure it out.*

But my initial bravado aside, I didn't have a clue how to do it. What I did know was that failure was no longer an option, like it had been so many times before. My job was on the line and I was not going to risk a high-profile TV gig simply because of my size. I knew I could fix this, despite having failed at every weight-loss plan ever invented. I told myself: *You cannot sentence yourself to a lifetime of whispers: "Tory was good on* Good Morning America, *but they got rid of her because she's fat."*

Besides, I needed to keep my job. Because I was the breadwinner in my family, the salary mattered. But I was also tired of the withering looks that all fat people get—the stares that say *you're lazy, weak, and undisciplined.* I would prove to everyone that I was none of those things and that what they saw on the outside hardly mirrored the strength I had on the inside.

That's exactly what I did.

Over the course of just one year, armed with a game plan, plenty of support from my family, and grit that I never knew I had, I did the unthinkable: I lost sixty-two pounds—the equivalent, as my son Jake puts it, of two Marlys, our thirty-pound beagle. How did I do it? For the first time, I shifted the way I viewed food—and myself. My story recounting that journey became *The Shift*, a book that resonated with thousands of women who had struggled forever with their weight. The best part? I haven't gained any of it back. In fact, I've shed a few more pounds. For me, there is no going back, just like a smoker or drinker who decides, finally, that enough is enough.

The response from readers has been my greatest gift: Women email me, stop me on the street, and corner me in shopping malls, supermarkets, and department stores to tell me that my story is their story and we must be sisters from another mother. Why is it, they ask, that so many diet books offer false hope and gimmicks instead of straight talk? They thank me for sharing a struggle that had always humiliated me—an uncomfortable topic that I never expected to share publicly. They say that reading about my challenges gave them the courage to make shifts in their lives, too.

After my Shift, I felt better about myself than I ever had before. I went to my doctor after avoiding having a physical for more than ten years because I hadn't wanted to be lectured about my size. Dressing rooms were no longer frustration destinations but places to explore the new me with clothes I had never thought would fit. I was a better role model for my kids, especially my teenage daughter, Emma. I embraced exercise, had more energy and enjoyed better sex, and became confident about my appearance for the first time ever. I genuinely valued all of the empowering things that came from losing weight.

But I also expected something more to happen.

I couldn't quite articulate what that was, but let me ask you this: Have you ever accomplished a goal only to discover, after all is said and done, that you feel empty? I had always thought *if only* I could lose weight, *everything* in my life would be *perfect*. I pretty quickly discovered that life doesn't work that way. Tackle one area and other stuff pops up. That's just the way life is, one big game of Whac-A-Mole. I didn't expect it, but that's what happened. I began to realize that I had attributed all the challenges in my life to being overweight and had convinced myself that once my weight was under control everything would be *perfect*. In some ways, everything *did* feel *perfect*—for a while. But before long my life began to unravel, or at least that's how it seemed. I had Shifted on the outside—and yes, on the inside too—but looking back, I wasn't really any different on the inside. I think I expected the whole world to stand up and take notice. I wanted some huge prize for losing the weight. Not a

Mirror Ball Trophy from *Dancing with the Stars* or a rose from *The Bachelor*. But something *big*. I figured I'd know it when it hit me. Then I waited and waited, but no prize arrived. No chariot pulled up with my reward. Rainbows and unicorns did not appear in the sky and neither did shooting stars and fireworks. Hope and expectation turned to disappointment and restlessness, which puzzled me because I had expected nothing but blue skies from now on. I was no longer obese, so why wasn't everything perfect? Why wasn't I so much happier?

Now, don't get me wrong. I lost all this weight and I continue to be thrilled with the results. I'm happy that I did it my way, that my willpower and determination paid off and that I didn't revert to old habits. But looking back, I put too much emphasis on the fictitious notion that a lower number on a scale would fix everything. If only I could lose forty, fifty pounds, I would get the recognition I deserved, phenomenal job opportunities would open up, motivational speaking engagements would pour in, and I'd be a kinder, gentler, less stressed-out version of Tory Johnson. Instead, I discovered that weight loss alone is not the be-all and end-all; size does not determine inner happiness. That was a massive letdown. I was clearly in a funk and I needed to figure out how to feel as good on the inside as I did on the outside. I wanted to experience the kind of inner satisfaction and contentment that couldn't be measured in numbers. I wanted to Shift the way I viewed and lived other parts of my life with the same determination I had used to lose weight.

I wanted to Shift for Good.

But that's easier said than done because Shifting the way you approach your life—and the way you feel about yourself, way down deep inside—is far different from Shifting the way you eat. I wasn't sure how I'd tackle it. I didn't have the luxury of taking a year off to travel—I can't even remember my last two-week vacation—and I certainly couldn't skip off to a Zen monastery to find myself. And while my curiosity is piqued when people ditch corporate careers to head to Caribbean islands to bartend on a beach, I have no interest in abandoning my life or the people in it.

I wasn't about to pack my bags, but I did want to explore this whole mind-body connection with the goal of becoming more content and even more familiar with who I am. My experiments in search of contentment had to be realistic for a working mom, a busy girl on the go, and they needed to be cost-effective. Low- or no-cost would be even better: I'm not known as the "Deals & Steals" lady on *Good Morning America* for nothing.

I wanted to build what I think is best described as a portable sense of self-esteem, one that would stay with me wherever I went, so that no matter what issues I faced, I wouldn't get rattled. My goal was to find ways to make me feel good about myself, the right tools and tactics to face challenges like job loss, financial hits, aging spouse, empty nest, or death, to name a few. I was desperate to calm the incessant chaos inside me. I yearned to be happy and healthy, inside and out.

So for the second time in my life, I had an honest conversation with myself. *Enough is enough*, I thought. *No more gimmicks. No more lies. No more excuses. You're a smart girl. Figure it out.*

And I did. I stepped out of my comfort zone and tried a bunch of new things with the same grit and determination that had served me well during my initial Shift. This time, I focused on what was happening on the inside, with an eye toward rethinking and re-imagining myself and how I wanted to lead my life going forward. *Shift for Good* is the story of how I learned to ride more waves instead of crashing onto the rocks—and how you can, too.

The Shift was a pretty straightforward journey for me: I went from fat to (fairly) fit. Initially I wrote that I had gone from "fat to fit," but changed it to include "fairly" because, truth by told, I am a work in progress. My friend Linda chastised me because we're all works in progress and that doesn't mean we can't celebrate who we are and our accomplishments, at this very moment, without apology or caveats. I will try to keep that reminder front and center.

Shift for Good takes a more circuitous path, and I experienced some hiccups along the way. Being more present, finding peace and joy and sharing them with people I love, continue to evolve. Appearing on *Good Morning America* each week makes me a familiar face to viewers. But I'm not a self-help guru, psychologist, or shrink. I'm just a woman with a happy family and a good career who found herself in a jam and needed to find a way out. As I did in *The Shift*, I embarked on a mission to figure it out for myself. In the following pages, I share candidly what I did. It's up to you to decide which parts might work for you. All I ask is that you keep an open mind, which is the one promise I made to myself going into this.

SHIFT
for GOOD

A NEW ME

Cheers to a new year and another chance for us to get it right.

—*Oprah Winfrey*

On Cloud Nine in the Land of Oz

t's October 22, 2013, a month after *The Shift* has hit bookstores, making its debut at No. 1 on the *New York Times* bestseller list—the Big Daddy of book charts and the dream of every author. What I'm about to do feels so good: I'm standing in the studios of *Dr. Oz*, ready to be introduced for a live segment. I'm wearing a size 6 cornflower blue J.Crew dress, a dramatic change from the size 16 pants that once dominated my bedroom closet without a single dress on any hanger. As a regular on *Good Morning America*, I know TV really well, but I'm blown away that I'm about to talk to Dr. Mehmet Oz, America's doctor. I'm very nervous.

I dreamed about this moment on the pages of *The Shift*, but now it's really happening. Because I've been The Fat Girl my entire life, my personal accomplishment coupled with the book's strong launch is a much-needed blast of sunshine. I feel like Sally Field when she accepted the Oscar for the 1984 movie *Places in the Heart*: "You like me! Right now, you like me!"

Barbara Fedida is here to cheer me on. She's the ABC News executive who started all this in the ABC cafeteria by suggesting that I see a stylist, which I instantly interpreted as *lose weight or else*. At a book party that she and the *Good Morning America* anchors threw for me at her East Side apartment days earlier, I described Barbara as The Velvet Dagger. She stuck it to me smoothly about my weight, just enough to start me on my healthy living path. "She told me what I needed to hear," I said with tears in my eyes to a room full of ABC News colleagues who had come to congratulate me. "Without Barbara I would never have made my Shift." I meant it. Had it not been for her, I would have continued to ignore my weight and find more excuses for not making the effort.

Judging from the emails I get from women all over the world who read my story, I struck a common chord in *The Shift*. Nakia, an overweight Pennsylvania mom with a special-needs daughter and son, read the book the day it came out and writes to me weekly to share her progress. "I hope you don't mind the intrusion," her first email said, "but I'm praying that continuing to talk to you will make me more accountable."

"It was a rough week at home, but a great one on the scale," Nakia said in her latest report. "I'm down two more pounds and I'm so proud that I am doing this *for me*." This is a big breakthrough for my pen pal; prior to reading *The Shift*, she says, she devoted so much time to caring for her kids that she left no time for herself.

I'm flattered that Nakia and many other women are Shifting with me, because I never intended to write this book. My weight has always been my hidden shame, my secret demon, something that I reserved for private conversations with my mom but nobody else—not even my closest friends. I hid my body under loose-fitting black clothes, always embarrassed by my size. I felt very uncomfortable being naked at any time, even in the dark with Peter, my husband. If anyone outside my tight circle wanted to engage me in any sort of healthy living stuff, I quickly changed the subject.

Six months into my Shift, *Good Morning America* weatherman Sam Champion turned to me during a segment and out of the blue asked, "Do I see a slimmer Tory Johnson?" I was stunned at his impromptu remark because this was my confidential challenge—I had shared no details of what I was doing to lose weight except with my immediate family. I couldn't wait for a commercial break. But over the next few days I got hundreds of comments from women who wanted to know, "How *did* you lose all the weight?" Initially I wrote back with general guidelines, but when the queries didn't stop, I decided that perhaps my story might also help others.

That's when I decided to share my journey.

I know that women are perpetually looking for ways to lose weight because I had been one of them. For my whole life, I was a textbook example of why diet secrets grace the covers of supermarket tabloids in the checkout lines: I was so desperate to reduce my size that any fad diet headline, no matter how far-fetched, lured me. It's no wonder the diet industry pulls in $60 billion a year and why network morning shows and daytime talk shows feature every weight-loss story imaginable. Women crave the tips and true-life tales. I know this from experience because I tried so many of the diets without success.

I'd already written six books, but they dealt with finding jobs, working from home, and starting a business. This was a marked departure for me. I had no idea whether the story of how I finally shed weight by dramatically changing the way I viewed and consumed food would sell. I just knew I wanted to help other women facing the same demon. But I never imagined my story would resonate as much as it did, garnering extensive media coverage and candid feedback from scores of readers. I was stunned when *Good Housekeeping* excerpted *The Shift* in a multi-page spread and when editors at *People* magazine found my story inspiring. In a nod to Kim Kardashian and Kanye West, whose exploits are regular fodder in *People*, I quipped on Facebook, "Move over, Kimye!"

My lifelong battle with weight became a touching segment on *Good Morning America*, and after a very supportive Robin Roberts interviewed me, thousands of viewers reached out. I was flooded with long, detailed, and poignant emails from women across the country. When they said that my story was their story, it was something that no one had ever said to me. I began to feel a bond with women that I'd never experienced before—one that I found deeply gratifying and rewarding.

I felt an obligation to women like Nakia: while I had their backs by reading their emails and responding to them personally, I also sensed that they had mine, too. Putting my story out there was my insurance against ever gaining back the weight: with so many women watching me every week on TV, there was no way I could let them down after I showed them a path to healthy living. I took none of their attention or emails for granted because I felt their pain and knew exactly what they're going through. We were in it together.

That I actually lost the weight, had the courage to write about it, and ended up with a bestseller was as good a trifecta as I could imagine. That I'm now about to talk about it on national television with Dr. Oz is an over-the-top bonus that has me almost pinching myself to see if it's real, just like Dorothy when she finally meets the Wizard.

Before I walk out on the stage, a two-minute taped piece tells my background story. Then Dr. Oz greets me in front of the applauding audience of women as though I'm Cinderella, the belle of the ball. "You look fabulous," he whispers, twirling me around, but loud enough so that the microphone picks it up. I mean, come on, way to make a girl swoon. It gets better when the two of us sit down to talk.

"You look absolutely marvelous!" he says as we sit down. He recalls reading the book on a plane. "It is so honest—painfully honest."

His vote of support means so much to me. When I respond that he's in it, he asks me to read the passage out loud. I explain to the audience that in the early pages of *The Shift*, I described my anxiety over the coming journey and making it to the finish line. Opening the book to the passage, I begin to read: *I envision myself on Dr. Oz's couch talking about my dramatic weight loss as women in the audience hang on my every word.*

I'm not sure if someone hit the APPLAUSE sign, but boy do they cheer. I talk about how happy I am to finally see my physician and learn that I am healthy. Oz nods in agreement when I admit that I avoided a physical for more than a decade: "I was ashamed of my weight and desperately wanted to avoid a lecture about it." Oz says white coat fear is especially high among overweight women and that physicians are partially to blame.

"I know how much we (doctors) embarrass women by asking them to get on scales," Oz says. "I learned that since I began doing the show because I did not appreciate that beforehand. The reason women don't go to the doctor is they don't want to see the numbers."

For a man who has seen it all when it comes to diets and knows every gimmick out there, he is impressed by tricks he's never heard of, ones that I use when the urge to eat hits me. "Painting my nails with top coat is the perfect way to avoid mindless snacking: it's impossible to eat anything with wet nails and the time the polish takes to dry is just enough to let my hunger pangs pass," I tell him. "A garlic pickle or two has zero carbs and zero calories and curbs my craving to eat bad things. There's something about those salty suckers that does the trick."

I also talk about the power of a photo. "Some women hang up cutouts of *Sports Illustrated* supermodels in bathing suits to inspire them to lose weight, but I knew I'd never look like Kate Moss or have a model's figure, so I did the opposite. I hung unflattering photos of my face with multiple chins on the refrigerator and put one on the wall near my desk to remind myself that those images were far from my best self."

Before I know it the audience is applauding again. It's over.

Oz gives me a peck on the cheek. Backstage, producers tell me it was a home run. My phone is lighting up with texts congratulating me on the appearance. I'm on Cloud Nine.

Few things feel as fabulous as finding your focus and knowing that you're on fire.

Losing My Shift

2

L iking those cupcakes, are you, Mommy?" my sixteen-year-old daughter, Emma, asks good-naturedly. She's about to lie on my bed and chat with me into the night, as she does so often. When I don't respond, she returns to her bedroom. I hear bits and pieces of her whispering to her twin brother, Jake: *Mom...bad...mood.* That doesn't begin to describe the darkness that envelops me right now, six months after my *Dr. Oz* lovefest.

I've wolfed down not one but two sugar-laden cupcakes, a treat from friends who spent the weekend with us. This is nervous eating-without-thinking-about-the-consequences behavior that has plagued me throughout my life. It is what made me fat. It always starts innocently enough: I take a dab of frosting and lick it off the tip of my finger. But then I take another dab and then another. Before I know it, I'm pulling back the paper and digging into the cake part. And then I do it all over again. It is something I haven't done, or even been tempted to do, since my Shift, when I swore off sweets.

Feeling sorry for myself after my cupcake gobble, I begin

10

reviewing a laundry list of personal and professional woes that have cropped up in the few months since the glow of *The Shift* has dissipated. My *Dr. Oz* appearance is long gone. So are the book signings, media interviews, and *Shift*-related speeches that buoyed me through the end of 2013. The festivities are distant memories and the incredible high I got from all the hoopla has given way to the ho-hum of ordinary days, which now seem chock-full of challenge.

The run-up to *The Shift*'s publication was an all-consuming process that left little time to focus on much else, including the core businesses I had started when my kids were babies. Then the rollout of the book sucked me in even more, right through to the extended victory lap. Nothing that lies ahead seems nearly as thrilling. I'm in a funk, which has triggered my little cupcake fest. It's the same mindless eating that I engaged in my whole life for comfort or escape, simply because it was an easy, pleasurable option.

It's natural to believe that when we do A and accomplish B, then we'll get C and be done. But more often than not, when we do A and accomplish B, unexpected things arise to delay C because, well, that's life and life is always an unpredictable journey. You think you'll (A) meet the right partner, (B) get married, and (C) live happily ever after. But after A and B, you're not really happy, because you want a baby. After years of trying, you give birth, but you're still not happy because you're forty pounds heavier and you can't seem to lose the weight. It's a whole lot harder than you thought it'd be. And you want more money. Your full-time job isn't nearly as exciting as it once was and you're desperate to find a better work-life balance with the baby and your spouse, too—the one you've been ignoring.

When I first Shifted, (A) I changed the way I viewed food and myself, and as a result (B) I lost a lot of weight, so (C) I expected to be happy forever. Game over. Yet here I am, a few months after the glow of *The Shift* has died down, by now a good seventy-plus pounds lighter but not a whole lot happier. In fact, I'm about to grab another cupcake.

My physical appearance has changed, but in many ways my life has stayed the same.

Emma's innocent teasing about the cupcakes jolts me back to reality. I cannot allow myself to ever return to the on-again/off-again eating treadmill because it's bound to end in disaster. I refuse to ever subject myself to stares from people who could see I had gained all the weight back. So, no more cupcakes for me.

Some of the zingers I got from women after I lost weight are still very fresh in my mind. No doubt they meant to be kind, but their comments came with an undercurrent of cruelty. One professional acquaintance, a small-business coach in central Florida who is obsessed with running and cycling, held me by both arms as she told me how happy she was for me: "I worried for so long because you had really let yourself go." A mommy blogger from Philadelphia congratulated me in an email by saying, "Since you're on TV, I'm sure you were ashamed of how you looked and now you don't have to be." I'm still not sure what these women meant to convey, but what came across, what I heard, was *"Now that you're 'normal,' we can finally tell you the truth about how disgusted we were with the way you looked."* I've let most of those insults slide off my back since I've won a great personal victory, but I do not forget them.

Now that the weight is gone, it occurs to me that there are

more layers in my life that I need to peel off and address—and that makes me uneasy. The truth is, I've lost the weight but I haven't lost my Fat Girl mentality, with all the insecurities and *poor me*s that accompany it. My feelings haven't shifted in any real meaningful way. It's not that my life isn't good. I have great kids, a loving husband and a rewarding career. But after the high of my accomplishment, I feel let down and I'm not sure why. I guess I imagined that once I lost the weight, life would be perfect—and it's not. It's yet another wake-up call.

Like many women who struggle with weight, I am well aware of what it feels like to use food as comfort to dull the pain, to temporarily ease every problem. I cannot start bingeing on food again if I want to have any chance of creating lasting change in my life and facing whatever problems arise in a more sustainable manner. In other words, I want to Shift for Good—not slide backwards.

"Liking those cupcakes, are you, Mommy?" is all I needed to hear to know that I can't allow food to soothe my woes ever again.

Just because your body changes doesn't necessarily mean your life will, too.

3

Woe Is Me

After the Cupcake Incident, I should be pleased that I was able to notice my old food-as-comfort behavior before it escalated into predictable pre-Shift patterns. But instead I see it as a sign of weakness. Indeed, a litany of personal and professional worries has consumed me lately and it bothers me that I am largely incapable of doing anything about them. Viewed separately, each might be manageable. But together they paint a portrait of emerging chaos in my life. In a nutshell, here's what's been going on.

Just months before *The Shift* hit bookstores, my very active, picture-of-perfect-health father went from diagnosis to death in just three weeks. His death from pancreatic cancer at sixty-six stunned family, friends, and colleagues who knew him as a prominent Miami architect who helped revitalize South Beach. But amid our grief comes a bigger surprise: two life insurance policies he had supposedly set up don't exist, which leaves my mother a shocked widow facing the unanticipated prospect of dramatically downsizing her lifestyle. I suddenly wonder if I'm going to have to support her at some point, a scenario that causes me some anxiety, especially since I'd do anything for my mom.

My father's death reminds me that my own husband is getting up in age. No matter how much I try to swat it away, I can't help but feel that Peter has suddenly gotten *old*. He is my rock, my best friend, my soul mate. When we married almost twenty years ago, I was just twenty-three and starting out while he was thirty-nine and divorced with two young children. He's still a kid at heart, quick as ever and the prankster he always was. But now he's about to turn sixty. His daughter, Tess, has just had a baby, which makes him a *grandfather*. Obviously there has always been a sixteen-year age gap between us, but still… sixty? That's a serious number, just five years from the legendary set-in-stone gold-watch retirement age. I still view myself as young: I have vivid memories of high school in Miami Beach and I'm just beginning to get used to no longer being in my thirties. How could this have happened so fast? How could my husband, now a grandpa, be approaching *sixty*?

Meanwhile my Grandma Evelyn, my mom's mom, is deteriorating. I suppose it's to be expected when you live to be eighty-nine, but she and I have always been close—I am her first grandchild—and it breaks my heart that Alzheimer's has begun to ravage her mind. Although she still recognizes my voice when I call—or else she does a remarkable job faking it—she has trouble remembering names and basic details, a sharp contrast to the witty and wise woman we all know and love. It's wrenching to watch her fade; harder still to realize that I'm powerless to stop it.

To top it off, as Jake and Emma prepare to enter their senior year of high school, the specter of an empty nest looms, and this saddens me the most. The life I've come to love is one with a house full of kids and their friends. For several years now, I've watched my twins leave in the summer to go off and do things that create great, lasting memories. But privately I dreaded sending them to sleep-away camp or on that life-changing monthlong trip to Ecuador to build a bridge in a rural village. Sure, Peter and I enjoy our time alone—we always click—and the silence that comes from not being constantly interrupted can be a welcome change.

But going off to college is different. It's the end of an era. Of course they'll return for breaks and vacations, but before long they'll seek more independence and value their time away from us, whether we like it or not. It's a fact of life that all parents face when their children leave the nest, but it still adds to my dis-ease.

Taken individually, none of these incidents is enough to run me off the rails, so to speak. I know logically that nothing I did has brought about any of these life-altering events. But coupled with what I perceive as pretty significant professional setbacks that have cropped up, they take their toll and threaten to undermine my newfound confidence.

To be perfectly honest, the whirlwind of activities that came along with *The Shift*'s incredible success got to my head because it was all so new and fresh and exciting. I daydreamed about becoming a nontraditional weight-loss guru, in demand for speeches. I relished my increasing visibility on *Good Morning America* "Deals & Steals," my weekly shopping segment, so much so that I spent my time looking at what might be possible with diet and deals to the detriment of my own women's career-focused businesses and the other aspects of my life.

In fact, based on the success of my "Deals" on *GMA*, other television producers approached me about expanding my role beyond that program. This was great news at first, because it felt like the prize I'd come to expect after losing all that weight. *I not only excel at my job, but I look great too!* Yet things didn't turn out the way I envisioned.

The producers were cautious by nature, so our discussions went on for months. With big money at stake, savvy executives, bean counters, and lawyers grilled me endlessly, questioning my assumptions, forecasts, methods, and goals. I spent countless hours laying the foundation, sourcing ideas, and crunching numbers.

There were times when I didn't think I could take another minute of the red tape. I'm not keen on corporate bureaucracy—the collective groupthink, cover-our-butts, stick-our-necks-out-for-no-one mentality, where committees seem to decide everything. But I played the game and went with the flow. For a couple of key in-person sessions, I spent hours in front of the mirror getting my hair and makeup just right.

Employing skills I learned as a high school debate champ, coupled with hard numbers and my proven success in the TV deals space, I'd managed to win over even the most skeptical execs. I was gratified that my hard work on "Deals & Steals" had been recognized and that I could now expand what I do to another fun show. Their lawyer had given me an eleven-page contract and both sides had at last agreed to wrap this up quickly so we could move ahead. The only things pending were our signatures.

When my phone rang, I answered with confidence and enthusiasm. I assumed this was a pro forma congratulatory call from one of the bigwigs who had been a strong advocate for me from our first meeting and an enthusiastic fan ever since. But instead she said, matter-of-factly, "We're withdrawing the offer and going in another direction. We like you a lot and this would've been a ton of fun. I'm so sorry it didn't work out."

The collapse of this deal, a really big deal, had me down. Big time. It depressed me because I was so sure it was a safe bet and didn't see the rejection coming at all. I was like any employee who can taste the promotion and assumes with confidence that it's all sewn up, only to be stunned when it doesn't happen. It made me feel very vulnerable and caused me to second-guess my normally reliable business radar, which had served me well for years.

We all know that disappointments like this occur frequently in every kind of business: internal plans change, bigger bosses weigh in, or things simply go in another direction. But no one expects it to happen to her—I certainly didn't. Privately, I had viewed this new deal as a reward of sorts for losing all the weight, perhaps even vindication for all the pain I had inflicted on myself by being obese for so long.

This is the part where I envisioned the payoff. *I lost the weight—now give me my prize.* It certainly didn't work out that way.

"You're like the girl who has been left at the altar—the bride who has planned this moment for months, if not longer, and she's even fantasized about her future blessings: the house, the lawn, the kids, a family—never in a million years expecting it to not happen," my friend Jodi says calmly over the phone. "When she's ditched, when she's all alone, she is embarrassed and betrayed, and the walls crumble."

"I think your analogy is too dramatic and I'm not sure it applies to me," I say defensively. But she is right: during my courtship with my would-be TV suitors, I didn't want to see—and I certainly didn't look for—any signs that this whole thing might go south. My ego got puffed up when I lost all the weight and *The Shift* did so well that I conflated that victory with effortless success in every area of life. I coasted on my laurels, viewing them as all-encompassing. I lulled myself into complacency, dreaming of only good things to come. The last thing I wanted to face were my ongoing, vexing worries.

My disappointment over the lost deal contributed to my spiral into the *poor me*s, which took a toll on my existing businesses. I was so convinced that I was destined for greatness that I neglected to notice (or even care about) the needs of my employees or the health of my company. Off in my own little world, I wasn't even concerned when three loyal members of the team gave their notice within a short time of one another. Instead of acting like the boss, I behaved like a petulant child when one of them, my most trusted aide, told me she was unhappy—maybe because it cut too close to the bone. *Unhappy? I spent forty years being unhappy because I was obese. I'll show you unhappy.*

So here I am, sitting on my bed as my laundry list of woes buzzes through my head like wasps in a nest. I'm in a daze, unable to concentrate on anything. From my bed, I stare at the large flat-screen TV on the dresser but I have no idea what program is on. I am feeling oh-so-sorry for myself. *Why does my life seem to be so unsatisfying and full of clouds? Why am I feeling so much blah? Why does my life suck?*

"In the span of a few months I've gone from the highest high to the lowest low," I tell Peter, as tears of frustration begin to flow. "So much of this is out of my control. I feel helpless and I hate that."

The box of Kleenex is next to me on my nightstand, but when I don't reach for it and let the tears run down my face, he comes over and hands me a couple of tissues. Peter has seen this weak, vulnerable, woe-is-me side before. As I dab my face he holds me tight and we lie there silently for a few minutes.

When I recover, he asks me to think back to the years when I was heavy and how what we've come to call "The Chat" with Barbara was all I needed to trigger my Shift. It was a pivotal time when I broke decades of bad habits and created a new life-style for myself, with virtually no input from anyone else.

He reminds me that I spent much of my life convinced that my weight was genetic and that I could never change my destiny. "But once you set your mind to it, you learned you had a lot more control than you ever believed you did," he says as we drift off to sleep. "I bet a lot of what you did then will help you now. You'll figure a way out this funk. I'm sure of that and I'm sure of you."

Peter's pep talk helped snap me out of my doldrums. I knew it was up to me to figure it out. I'd have to banish my inner Fat Girl once and for all.

Sometimes when you're down, there's no place to go but up.

Fat Forever

4

On *Good Morning America*, I'm Tenacious Tory, quick on her feet and oozing self-confidence as the "Deals & Steals" gal who offers great bargains on products. I'm also the "jobs lady" who discusses career and workplace issues with the broadcast's anchors. I do all of that in addition to running my own companies, which I founded fifteen years ago. You don't get on national TV or become a successful entrepreneur by being a wallflower or letting others determine your destiny.

But behind my can-do façade there is Timid T, a vulnerable girl whose weight still haunts her. *The weight that is no longer there.* Yes, I've lost more than seventy pounds by now, but when I look in the mirror, I still see The Fat Girl. She is my albatross.

For most of my life, no matter how hard I tried, I was incapable of being anything other than a plus-size woman. There came a depressing point, after I had failed at yet another fad diet, when I became resigned to my fate: I was destined to be large and there was nothing I could do about it. I learned how to use clothes to camouflage my weight (or at least I thought I did).

Borrowing tricks from makeup artists, I learned how to contour my cheekbones in order to look thinner. And of course, on those rare occasions when I allowed myself to be photographed for professional or personal reasons, I insisted the photo be taken from a certain angle. Photoshop became my best friend.

I was a compulsive eater and carb junkie for forty years. From the minute I was able to chew solid food, my go-to picks were rice, pasta, bread, chips, cakes, and candy bars. The higher the carb count, the better. My mom stuffed our freezer with ice cream and pizza rolls. We rarely used the bottom oven of our stove because it housed Funyuns, Oreos, Chips Ahoy!, nacho-cheese-flavored Doritos, Ruffles potato chips, Cheetos, and Cheez-Its. Kids came over and made a beeline for the oven, and so did I—many times a day.

When I was seven, my mom sat me down on the brown velour couch in the living room, and announced she was pregnant. The thought of having another sibling, a real baby in the house, thrilled me. We celebrated the good news that night at McDonald's. I had a kid's meal: hamburger, fries, and a Coke—one of thousands of poor food choices I would make in the coming decades. By second grade I was already twenty pounds overweight. In class pictures, I'm The Fat Girl. I had a normal metabolism and my adrenal glands worked fine. I was fat because I ate too much and was hooked on sugar.

After many failed efforts to dodge phys ed class at Treasure Island Elementary School and then at Nautilus Junior High, I made it to Miami Beach Senior High determined to never don a pair of gym shorts again. I forged a letter from my mom saying I had a back injury, and it worked: my gym days were finally over. Throughout high school the most exercise I got was lifting a cookie to my mouth, turning the key to my convertible, or walking to and from it. In parking lots I cruised around until a spot opened up near where I was going. At home, I lay on the couch.

As is the case in many families, food was comfort. Good day? Celebrate with an entire bag of Cool Ranch Doritos. Bad mood? Have a frozen microwave pepperoni pizza. Depressed? Let this box of Entenmann's chocolate chip cookies cure it. I drank sugared soda with abandon. When I thought of a "healthier" drink choice, I opted for fruit juices, oblivious to calories, sugar, or carbs. I was a Florida Citrus Growers dream: I viewed anything with fruit as healthy and never considered it as liquid sugar—Tropicana orange juice, Ocean Spray cranberry, Welch's grape juice, those little shiny Capri Sun packages.

All of this was happening in the late 1970s and early '80s, hardly the Dark Ages. America's fitness craze was catching on. People joined health clubs, took up jogging, and in Miami Beach, where I lived, wore as little as possible, flaunting six-pack abs and rocking their bikinis. But in our house we never talked about any connection between calories and obesity. Nor did we stop to wonder about healthier food options or link our food choices to our expanding waistlines.

My parents both worked and came home tired. Neither had much interest in cooking or whipping up complicated meals. Dinner prep often fell to me and since I was a kid, the easier the better. I became an expert at making packaged meals like Hamburger Helper, scalloped potatoes, and Rice-A-Roni. I fried hot dogs and hamburgers and created puddles of grease. Every meal included rice, baked potato, or pasta. No one in my family ever complained. Who doesn't like that stuff?

Flora's was a popular outdoor pizzeria in Miami, and once a week we headed there for garlic knots and pepperoni pies. We stopped often at a local bakery for fresh corn muffins and my favorite: chocolate cream-filled hi-tops.

One day, during a routine appointment, my dentist asked Mom if she was "gaining or expecting," as if he were asking about the weather. My mother, beautiful and stylish in my eyes then and now, was not pregnant: at that point my brother, David, was already three. She and I never acknowledged the dentist's cruel comment. Instead, we went to Carvel for soft-serve ice-cream cones.

Unlike David, a chubby kid who became ripped in college, I never managed to lose the childhood blubber on my thighs, butt, or belly. I hated being fat and tried many times to lose weight, but throughout my twenties and into my thirties I failed at one diet after another. By my early forties I began to accept that I'd never change, and in some ways I made peace with it—at least that's what I told myself. But I never did: I was ashamed of my size and wanted desperately to look "normal." I resented the looks I got because of my weight, and I wanted nothing more than to crawl into a secret place and hide. Yet at the same time I was desperate for a way out. Such is the life of The Fat Girl.

Finally, after The Chat with Barbara, I felt I had one last chance: I would solve this weight riddle once and for all.

I knew I needed to lose weight, but I'd be damned if I'd go on a *diet*. After years of yo-yoing, I had finally concluded that diets are temporary pauses in bad behavior. Even the phrase *going on a diet* implies temporariness because the flip side is *going off*. No, I decided, what I needed was a permanent lifestyle change and not a set of prescribed rules or gimmicks that promise outrageous results in a few days or weeks. That's the stuff of all fads. None of them work long-term and I was done with them. This time, I would carve out a plan that I could live with and take with me no matter where I was, one that would be mine forever.

I knew that it would require a cognitive shift in the way I viewed eating and food, and that what I put in my head and the stories I told myself would be far more powerful than anything I put in my mouth. I vowed to stop fooling myself with bogus reasons like *this is a bad day, or month, or year to start eating healthy*. Or *the holidays are coming so what's the use*, when I knew very well it was July and that Thanksgiving and Christmas were months away.

I learned to forgive myself, to ditch the habit of using any setback as an excuse to lose momentum and return to eating bad stuff. I embraced the power of the pause and found that taking a walk around the block, doing an errand, or layering on another coat of clear nail polish often diverted my attention from my empty stomach long enough to keep me from making a poor food choice. Working my willpower muscle took practice, but over time it became strong, very strong. There were times when I gave in to temptation and cheated. But instead of caving and abandoning my plan like I used to when I'd fall off the wagon, I got back on that horse again—immediately, the same day.

I remember vividly being in full Shift mode a few days before Easter 2012, when I walked into a Target store in Edgewater, New Jersey. In front of me was my all-time favorite sugary delight: a full display of those little Cadbury chocolate-coated

Easter eggs. I had always anticipated the arrival of Cadbury mini packs during the weeks preceding the holiday. Sure, it would have been okay to eat one little pack. But I never did. I'd scarf down the whole giant grab bag, twelve servings or so, without thinking about the consequences. They're small, I figured, so I'd keep popping them in my mouth. Yum.

But this time I wasn't tempted at all. I felt like an alcoholic whose life had been turned upside down by booze and now hated the stuff and wouldn't ever touch it again. It was a major victory for me to realize that I could stare at that sweet delight without reaching toward the shelf. It was there, right in front of me, but I could walk away—and I did.

A few months after *The Shift* was published, I delivered a speech in Washington, D.C. to a group of event planners about the personal and professional shifts we make in life. When I opened it up to questions, one woman told me that she had tried and failed many times to lose weight. When I asked her why she'd failed so often, she said she really couldn't figure it out. I prodded her a little more, asking if she followed a strict meal plan with no cheating. She admitted she had a serious weakness for pretty much any type of fast food. "In all honesty," she asked, "how did you get to the point where you were okay with never again treating yourself to an order of French fries?"

"Fuck the fries," I blurted out. "Focus on the dress." After the laughter died down, I explained that a key lesson I'd learned during my Shift was that I had to embrace the concept of all-or-nothing.

"If you're really committed to losing weight, nothing can trump your resolve," I told them. "One fad diet after another says that if you're good for six days, you can eat anything you want on the seventh—as a reward. But I wasn't born with the moderation gene." I went on to say that cheat days for me are akin to giving an alcoholic a beer or two to celebrate a month of sobriety. It doesn't work. A carbo load can't be a reward for healthy eating because all it does is get me off track and on to eating crap again. Heads nodded when I equated my former eating habits with other addictions and explained that a cigarette after a month of not smoking does more harm than good to the person determined to kick the habit.

I told the group that I had spent so much of my life obsessing about food, about every little fry. And if it wasn't fries, it was something else. "Are my six days up yet? When can I get my hands on the next cupcake? What flavor will it be? Will I eat the icing before the cake part? What if I want more than one?"

Peter often encourages me not to be so hard on myself. He reminds me that one bite isn't the end of the world. For many people, that's true. But my truth is that I can't handle moderation. "Just one bite" often doesn't stop there. Then boom—the scale is my truth teller. One bite leads to so many more. In a flash I'm back to reality—my reality—that I wasn't born with the moderation gene. For me, avoidance is better than attempting moderation. I remind myself that it's so much more satisfying to indulge in stuff that's good for me instead. My latest craze is zucchini "noodles" with meat sauce as a substitute for pasta.

Thanks to that one question, my time with the event planners evolved into a quasi-Weight Watchers, true-confessions session. I wrapped things up by saying, "I had to stop obsessing over fries and imagine zipping up a fitted dress so I could show up at an event with confidence, instead of hiding under oversize clothing and staying home. Isn't that more meaningful than any potato?"

I feel good about my weight now and I know there's no going back to my old ways. Not a chance. But I want to figure out how to stop being The Fat Girl and banish the voice inside my head that keeps telling me I'm not worthy, that I'll always struggle, that I'll never be happy. I need to replace my inner Fat Girl with an inner certainty that matches the confidence I exude outwardly. Just as I did with food, I need to carve out a plan that will allow me to Shift for good, that I can take with me no matter where I am, that will be mine forever.

I'm not naïve enough to believe there won't be challenges along the way. Of course there will. And, while much of this funk is self-imposed, I trace a lot of it back to my work ethic and the stress I put on myself to be perfect.

When Peter wrote for *USA Today*, a job he held for most of his thirty-one-year newspaper career, he used to tell me that he was only as good as his last column. "It doesn't really matter how many balls I hit out of the park today because readers and my bosses expect a new column tomorrow," he'd say. "And they want a new one the next day, too. It's one of those jobs where you have to prove yourself each and every day."

I feel the same way with my TV segments and career events. There's a natural tendency on the part of people who see you performing well to expect a better performance the next time, and the next time after that. The bar is always being raised. We all want to deliver really great work, but it can be extremely demanding and exhausting. Each women's career event I host has to be better than the one before. When I deliver a terrific "Deals & Steals" segment, topping it the next time is tough. And if I manage to do that, am I really expected to top that, too? In some ways, the answer is yes. When you play in the big leagues, the stakes are high, along with the standards, and much is expected, as well it should be.

In many ways, the pressures I face pale in comparison to what many others confront day in and day out. In sports, you're only as good as your last at-bat. Actors and singers are held to the highest standards on their latest album, play, or movie. Sales professionals must outperform their previous numbers. We judge others that way, and it's how I've come to judge myself.

Peter's been pretty sick of my whole attitude lately, to put it mildly. "Your outlook sucks and you seem to have checked out. I don't like seeing you this way, not for me and not for our family. I'm tired of the way you've been treating me." Peter isn't easily bothered and he can put up with a lot, so it's rare for him to come down hard on me. Listening to the seriousness in his voice and seeing the pained look on his face, I know that I've pushed beyond the limits.

"I'm here to help and support you," he says, "But you're the one who must figure this out before you dig yourself and all of us into an even deeper hole."

My pity party is over. I am going to figure out how to end this once and for all. To do that, I have to delve a little deeper. But how?

I was never into any kind of New Age stuff: all that spirituality and holistic hooey were far too touchy-feely for me. But my friend Heidi has been an avid booster of all forms of self-help for years, from attending multi-day Tony Robbins retreats to whole-body cryotherapy, in which you spend two to three intense minutes exposing your body to freezing nitrogen gas. It seems like each week I get a breathless call from her saying, "I just came back from [fill in the blank]—you must try this!" The calls seemed so insistent and the schemes so out there, so woo-woo, that I had trouble taking any of it seriously and pretty much dismissed the entire genre.

But now I can see that perhaps I was a little too quick to judge. Case in point: Five years ago I participated in a fire walk at a small-business retreat outside Dallas. In a fire walk, hot coals are placed in a path and you walk barefoot across it to prove your inner strength and courage. It's no joke, which is why firemen with hoses stand by in case anything goes wrong. Prior to the walk, I dismissed it as a mind-over-matter stunt, but to this day women who did it with me still talk about how memorable and empowering the experience was. "If I can walk on fire and not get burned, I can do anything" was a common refrain in our group.

Obviously not everyone shares my skepticism about the self-help industry, as evidenced by its enormous popularity. But I do know that I'm not the only one who questions its legitimacy. Some women view practices designed to make them feel more content or increase their happiness quotient as trendy or gimmicky. They think all that "finding inner peace" stuff is for the ladies-who-lunch crowd: women with too much time on their hands.

But the truth is we all want to be happy and we owe it to ourselves to figure out the best ways to make that happen. By dismissing a lot of self-help techniques with one broad stroke, I now realize that I essentially ruled out practices that could have helped me relax and feel better about my life all along. I had to learn the hard way that sleeping in, getting a manicure, taking long showers, or luxuriating in a hot bath surrounded by candles and soft music could take me only so far. What it couldn't do was help me to feel as good about my inner self as I did about my outer self. In the meantime, I reckoned I wasn't crazy and an occasional neck massage was good enough. Or so I thought.

Nothing I've done so far has stopped me from being stressed-out, feeling like I could lose it at any moment, living in a constant state of self-doubt, or any number of things that come with being a busy woman. Maybe it's the wisdom that busy women face. Maybe I've finally woken up. But I get it now: My state of mind matters. A lot.

I no longer fantasize about telling millions of *Dr. Oz* viewers how I lost the weight. Instead, I'm in *Super Soul Sunday* mode, craving the chance to embark on a mental journey that I'll share someday with Oprah and her audience. I can picture myself admitting that my assumption about what real happiness is—losing seventy pounds—actually prevented me from getting there. And I'll go on to say, with complete conviction, that getting to the top of my weight-loss mountain and staying there would have been a heck of a lot easier if I had done the inner work first. Sure, losing weight made me a lot happier than I was, but now I realize that lasting happiness and contentment can't be sustained through a single accomplishment. Whatever that accomplishment is, it's only one slice of the pie—the non-edible kind, of course. I must focus on all pieces of my life: I want to honor my relationships, create a healthier connection between my body and my mind, be financially successful, give back to others, foster a calm environment, and stay curious and playful. I sense tackling all of those areas—and nurturing them consistently—is the ticket to lasting joy.

None of us can live thinking it'll never rain or that we'll never get caught in a downpour. But we can protect ourselves from getting swept away by the storm. Learning to manage stress levels and to trust my own inner guidance will help me stay grounded and feel more content every day. My quest will no doubt lead to some dead ends, but it'll be worth it if I'm left with the right tools and tactics in my mental health toolbox. I want to make "happy calm" the norm in my life, not the exception; I want to explore new ideas and practices with an eye toward living a better, less harried life. In the chapters ahead, I share my path toward inner peace; walk along with me and see if any of my suggestions and experiences resonate with you.

When you're at a point where the pain of the present outweighs the pain and sacrifice that change demands, you're ready to Shift for Good. The first key step in any Shift is getting fed up, desperately wanting something different for yourself, and knowing that change is your only option. That's where I am right now.

I'm ready to *Shift for Good.*

What you put in your head is far more powerful than what you put in your mouth.

FINDING INNER PEACE

We don't realize that, somewhere within us all,
there exists a Supreme Self who is eternally at
peace.

—*Elizabeth Gilbert*

5

Discovering Acupuncture

As I begin my quest, my biggest priority is to learn how to relax. I'm a driven Type-A woman and I've never really thought much about the importance of calming down. Incredibly, a few weeks after my Kleenex meltdown with Peter, I find my first way to chill literally next door.

As Peter and Marly stand in front of the elevator, outside our office, the doors open and a woman of a certain age gets off. Looking a bit confused, she asks, "Is this the fourth floor?"

"Yes, ma'am," Peter says.

"Who is this sweet angel?" she asks.

"This is Marly, the Prince of Eighty-Sixth Street," Peter answers.

She bends to pet him and seems ready to cry. "I had a beagle once, but they stole him."

Peter reaches out to comfort her, but suddenly she's all business. "Roberta Flack," the pop icon says by way of introduction as she extends her hand. Every day, radio disc jockeys still play her beloved hit single, "Killing Me Softly with His Song." For anyone who came of age in the 1970s, as Peter did, that is a defining song.

Our office is on the fourth floor of a decidedly unglamorous building that is home to a popular shoe store that serves everyone from toddlers to seniors. The faded ceiling tiles are laced with water stains and the uneven gray linoleum on the hallway floor is chipped in several spots. It was probably installed when "Killing Me Softly" was a Top Ten hit in 1973, maybe earlier. Peter, stunned to see a superstar there, asks what has brought her to his floor.

"Dr. Chang," the songstress says bluntly, pointing to suite 401, the office next to ours. "I wouldn't still be singing without him." High praise, Peter thinks.

Joseph Chang is a Chinese medical doctor and acupuncturist who had moved from another office uptown a few weeks earlier. Roberta lives two blocks to the east at the famed Dakota—the landmark building where Roberta's neighbor Yoko Ono, John Lennon's widow, has remained since he was shot to death there in 1980. That's Manhattan, where a dumpy office can sit within a stone's throw of a building where apartments go for millions of dollars.

Peter is intrigued. Maybe the drain of dealing with me and my moods, or simply his inquisitive nature, drives him to make an appointment. But the next thing I know, Peter is seeing Joseph regularly. After each visit he returns reporting that Joseph says he's stressed and needs to learn how to relax.

"*You* need to relax?" I laugh, incredulous. If anyone in our house has reason to be stressed, I think, it is me, myself, and I.

"He says too much stress is not healthy," Peter replies, ignoring the jab. "In fact, when I told him what happened to your dad, and how driven he was, he wasn't surprised. He believes strongly that stress contributes to cancer. He doesn't mince words about it."

Joseph teaches Peter a form of Tai Chi morning exercises, variations on the routines people do to kick-start their days in his native Taiwan. Jake and Emma start to find their dad in shorts each morning, floating his arms up and down, breathing in and out slowly, and rubbing various parts of his body in front of our large living room mirror. At night he listens to classical music with headphones on and eyes closed. After only a few acupuncture sessions, Peter begins to savor the benefits of the five-thousand-year-old practice of sticking tiny needles into body parts to cure whatever ails you.

"I feel like I've taken a Valium after I see him," Peter says. When a developing cold disappears overnight after just one session, Peter is hooked on the healing powers of traditional Chinese medicine and acupuncture. "I can't believe I've ignored this my whole life."

I know absolutely nothing about acupuncture, let alone Chinese medicine. And truth be told, I had always assumed it was a gimmick, if not some sort of scam. But every time we bump into her in the elevator or hallway, Roberta seems happy to see us, happier to see Marly, and happiest of all after her sessions with Joseph. I'm intrigued by Peter's and Roberta's testimonials, and one day when Peter says that Joseph has an opening, I'm ready to dive in and see him.

"Will I have to take off my clothes?" I ask Peter, cutting quickly to a sad and shameful by-product of being overweight most of my life: I'm still not comfortable with my naked body. I'm finally good with going to my doctor since I'm no longer in danger of getting a lecture about my size. And I love being able to wear dresses and all kinds of outfits that in my pre-Shift days would have looked comical. But I'm not sure I'm ready to face another professional who has a derobing requirement.

"You take off your outer clothes, but you're not naked and he gives you a big white oversize towel to cover yourself before he starts," Peter says. "He's extremely discreet and professional. Besides, I'll be seven feet away and you can scream for me."

The next afternoon I find myself in Joseph's studio. He is seated at a small white desk that seems more appropriate for a child. I am in front of him, sitting in a basic black metal folding chair, the kind you might find in a high school cafeteria. A privacy screen to my left separates his office from a massage table where he works on patients. For about fifteen minutes I fill out a surprisingly detailed medical history. Then Joseph takes my pulse in both wrists and examines my tongue with a bright halogen penlight, two basic diagnostic techniques that play a role in Chinese medicine. He does that with every patient during each visit.

"You think too much," Joseph says in heavily accented English, in a direct but nonjudgmental way. "You are excessively thinking."

I resist laughing in his face. *Thinking too much?* I mean, how many driven New Yorkers or Type A people might that apply to? And yet he's right: I *do* think too much. My mind races at lightning speed, a jumble of random ideas and musings and worries that seem to blend into a bowl of mental mush. Letting steaming hot water pour over my head every morning during my long shower helps only so much: my mind always seems to be operating at warp speed. Like my weight, I assumed there was nothing I could do about it.

Based on what his examination has revealed, Joseph tells me he's going to stick needles in a variety of places in my body, from my head to my feet. Over his right shoulder is a poster showing a schematic of a human body that explains the meaning of each spot or pressure point in Chinese medicine. *Needles?* I know Peter told me that's what acupuncturists do, but I hate needles. And where exactly does Joseph plan to stick them? How can poking needles in a needle-phobic woman make her feel more relaxed? I begin to wonder if I've made a mistake and if it's too late to bolt out of there.

Yet now I'm too chicken to change my mind. I am wearing a black V-neck T-shirt and jeans, which I keep on, but I remove my shoes and lie faceup on his table. Thankfully his technique is quick, professional, and virtually painless: He rubs a spot on my skin to warm it for a second before tapping a sterile needle into it. I wince only once or twice, but it's minimal, which says a lot coming from me. Over the course of fifteen minutes, Joseph taps nearly ninety needles into my face, hands, and feet. He focuses on precision, not speed, but he's very efficient. All I can think about is my face. What if, when he removes the needles, I'm left with a slew of red dots where the needles used to be? Will they fade away quickly or create scabs? Oh well, too late for that concern.

"Okay, thirty minutes. Be very still," he says, going around the screen to his side of his twenty-foot office. I'm not about to move—I don't want the needles to jiggle—and within a few minutes my eyes close and I am relaxed, not a care in the world.

This is My Time. There is nothing else, literally nothing, and I lie fully at rest, in this weird limbo between sleeping and waking. No conversation. No phone. No gum chewing. There's nothing but stillness. I could get used to this, I think.

I can't remember the last time I didn't wonder who was texting, emailing, or calling me; I'm always focused on all of that. But not now. This is total and complete relaxation. Why didn't I know about this twenty years ago, or even two years ago? My time with Joseph stands in stark relief to all that's happening outside, the fire trucks and ambulances routinely screaming by on our busy block. His table is next to a window overlooking the street, but with the blinds drawn and soft classical music playing, I tune out the ambient street noise without much effort. After a half hour, the time he says it takes for the human blood supply to make a round and refresh itself, Joseph removes the needles quickly, within a minute or so. He applies a cool paper mask infused with some sort of herbal potion on my whole face, except my nostrils.

The main aim of this session, he says, is to enable me to relax. "Bonus," he adds, is to brighten and lift my eyes. "Eyes are the soul," he tells me. He returns every few minutes to reapply various lotions to the mask, but I'm largely oblivious to what he's doing. I leave feeling refreshed and proud that I tried something new. For the rest of the day, I feel so good about myself that I don't bother putting on any makeup, something that's rare for me. And, for the record, no sign of needle marks anywhere— not a red dot in sight.

I do a fun segment on national television every week, but aside from that I like to think I'm a fairly normal woman. And from all the women I've met in my life, I know that many of us pay far more attention to others at the expense of our own self-care. When the yellow air masks drop from the ceiling of the plane, we look for someone else to help before we help ourselves. Big mistake. There is a reason why the flight attendants tell passengers to put the mask on themselves first.

The first thing I learned when I made my Shift was that eating well is oxygen. Then I learned that exercise is oxygen, too. Now, instead of looking to help someone else or ignoring my own needs, I am willing to admit that self-care is also oxygen. A healthier me is more equipped to help the people I love when they need it.

After just a few sessions, I now believe that acupuncture is the real deal and I'm a bit ashamed that I had dismissed it for so long. Prior to seeing Joseph, I would have claimed to be too busy to have time for such stuff. Now I get that I *have* to create time to care for myself. I've come to realize that deep relaxation, like I experience in acupuncture, calms my mind enough that I become more present and less reactive. When I'm on that table I can disconnect from my inner want demon (the one who thought life would be all rainbows and unicorns when I finally dropped the weight) and rediscover that part of me that knows true happiness comes from connectedness, service, and laughter.

While it's not realistic for me to see Joseph daily, I schedule a session every other week and acupuncture becomes one of the tools in my emerging self-care tool kit. Just knowing that these sessions are coming, that they are a permanent part of my routine, helps keep things in balance. I will no longer wait until I am in freak-out mode to do something for myself.

If you haven't tried acupuncture, I suggest you consider it. There are more than eighteen thousand licensed acupuncturists in the United States. Some health plans cover a series of visits. Ask friends if they have a practitioner they like, or simply research acupuncturists in your area. If cost is a factor, check to see if your city has a community acupuncture clinic, which allows patients to pay according to their means.

Be still and allow your energy to flow.

Finding Relief Through Meditation

T he stars at *Good Morning America* are pros, the best in the business. Robin Roberts, George Stephanopoulos, Lara Spencer, Amy Robach, and Ginger Zee all have their particular strengths. But as the face of ABC News, George is first among equals. He's the go-to guy viewers see for breaking news and all major events.

For the past five years George has practiced Transcendental Meditation. He doesn't preach about it, but he doesn't hide it either. He believes it has made a major impact in his busy life.

"I think people don't really understand exactly what it is and what a difference it's made in people's lives," George says during an on-air segment with his friend Jerry Seinfeld, who has been meditating for more than forty years, and the man who taught them both, Bob Roth. "What it really does is try to get the stress out of your life."

"You know how I describe it?" Jerry asks. "You know how you have a charger for your phone? TM is like having a charger

43

for your mind and body.'" Scientists are discovering the health benefits of meditation, Bob says, and the American Heart Association has found that TM is highly effective in reducing high blood pressure. He cites a *Forbes* magazine article that called stress the Black Plague of the modern era. "Stress is an ugly thing that can't be cured or prevented by conventional means, but this technique is highly effective in relieving it."

As I continue on the path toward wholeness, I want what they have. I want something I can lean on every day and do by myself, something that doesn't cost anything—much like jogging for runners. I'm not alone in my desire to learn meditation—*Psychology Today* says that more than ten million Americans do it—and my ABC News colleague Dan Harris wrote a bestseller about meditation called *10% Happier: How I Tamed the Voice in My Head, Reduced Stress Without Losing My Edge, and Found Self-Help That Actually Works—A True Story.* Dan is very vocal about how it turned his hectic life around.

Like I said before, until I began seeing Joseph Chang, one of the main ways (correction: the *only* way) I relaxed was by letting hot water stream down my face in the shower for fifteen minutes in the morning. And while I see Joseph regularly, I still feel that I need something that I can do every day on my own. Meditation, I think, could be a game changer for me.

So I make an appointment to see Bob, who runs the David Lynch Foundation in Manhattan. The calm begins from the moment I set foot in the reception area at the foundation's midtown offices. David Lynch, the famed director (*Eraserhead, Blue Velvet, Twin Peaks*), started his foundation in 2005 to teach TM to any kid who wants to learn. "The thing about meditation is you become more and more you," he once said. Now his group teaches TM to people everywhere, from underserved communities and veterans to Wall Street and media hotshots.

I once would have rejected meditation out of hand, just as I did acupuncture: touchy-feely malarkey practiced by holistic nuts with far too much time on their hands. But that's before I learn that George practices it in the wee hours, like 3 a.m., before heading to *Good Morning America* and then again in the evening. I respect his unflappable, calm-under-pressure demeanor. He is a steady man, so there must be something to this meditation stuff.

It's raining hard on the long wooden tables and the chairs on an outdoor deck. What a great day to be inside, I think, perfect for learning something that by all accounts should help me lead a more peaceful life. A framed quote on the wall reads *Change begins within.* Such a simple three-word sentence, yet it resonates deeply with me. Waiting to see Bob, I stare at the words and think about what has brought me here today: I am as determined as ever to change myself inside, and this is an essential step on that path. On the end table next to me is a reprint of an article from *GQ.* The title: "The Totally Stressed-Out Man's Guide to Meditation." This semi-stressed-out woman slips a copy into her handbag.

A few minutes later I'm seated in front of Bob in his airy, softly lit office. Speaking in a calm voice, he starts by saying that most people have some degree of skepticism about this ancient meditation technique called TM. "It's perfectly normal," he says matter-of-factly, which disarms me because he is saying exactly what I'm thinking: *of course* I'm skeptical. How can sitting still for 20 minutes at a time make that much of a difference? And anyway, it doesn't sound relaxing to me, it sounds uncomfortable. He continues: "You can be one hundred percent skeptical and still get the benefits of TM, just as you can be one hundred percent skeptical about how electricity works and still get the benefits from turning on a light switch." That makes sense. I have absolutely no clue how electricity works but I really like it and rely on it. And I like the way Bob explains things.

Over the course of the morning, he teaches me the basics of TM. He assures me that it's a technique, not a religion. It involves sitting in a chair and reciting a silent mantra to attain a state of relaxation. That alone is a news flash to me: You don't have to sit on a yoga mat, legs crossed, in a specific place, say OM or any of that stuff of TV or movie parodies. Whew. He gives me a simple-sounding, two-syllable mantra and urges me to not share it. This is mine and mine alone. Sharing with someone who hasn't been taught the basics, he says, puts too much emphasis on the mantra as the secret weapon. I'm perfectly willing to follow that honor code. I want to give this process my all.

Bob guides me with step-by-step instructions for several minutes and then asks me a few questions about what I felt. I don't think that I'm doing it right. That's normal, he tells me, which is why people who want the genuine benefits of proper meditation seek some form of training. Like many novices, I went into this thinking meditation is about clearing your mind. *Not* thinking. Having *no* thoughts. Zoning out completely.

But meditation is not about that; it's about getting the active brain settled. "None of us can stop thinking," Bob tells me, as if such a thought is preposterous. "Our brains aren't wired that way. Thoughts are perfectly normal."

I'm relieved to hear this because not only does my mind never stop, it seems to run in perpetual overdrive. I often worry that I'm going to burn out, which has made finding a reliable way to calm my mind a priority.

Bob has been meditating twice a day for more than four decades. I tell him I worry that I'll do it for a bit while it's new and fresh, then slack off once the novelty is gone. He says that's not uncommon, but that it probably won't be a concern once I begin to feel the benefits. "You don't forget to have coffee in the morning and you don't need any reminder: you just have it," Bob says, clearly speaking my language. "That's what happens when you get into meditation. The benefits are so profound that the practice becomes part of your day."

With consistency this soon becomes a habit: meditating twenty minutes in the morning and twenty at night is all it takes, he says.

Over the next few days I return to Bob's office for hour-long sessions to drill deeper and learn more. His colleague downloads an app on my phone, a simple meditation timer that he presets for twenty minutes, followed by a two-minute grace period to signal me to slowly come out of it. During the first couple of sessions I open my eyes often to peek at the time because twenty minutes feels like an eternity. Except for acupuncture sessions, I never stay completely still while awake. But unlike acupuncture, meditation has no needles that keep me in place. It's all on me. By Day Three of seeing Bob for what will be my sixth full meditation, I tell him that I've stopped looking at the time. I now want to take advantage of the full twenty minutes. I'm in no hurry for the gentle chimes that indicate time's up.

I ask if there's an increased benefit from extending that time. No, he says. Does it matter if the lights are on or off? No, as long as you're comfortable. All of this is music to my ears because it seems so doable.

I begin to meditate before I leave for work in the morning and after dinner. I find that I can do it even if Emma and Jake are talking loudly in another room, Peter is banging around the house, or Marly is moving about. Everyone can be doing their own thing and I can tune them out. I fluff up the pillows on my bed to prop myself up. Usually I'm in any old tee and my favorite well-worn sweatpants. It's simple and satisfying.

I don't trust myself to "find time" to practice twice a day. It's too easy to make excuses or simply forget. Instead I schedule my morning and night sessions on my calendar, treating them as I do every important commitment in my life. This is *my* time, as important to me as my food choices. Now, no matter where I am, whether I'm at home or on the road, I know how to recharge, just as Jerry Seinfeld does. And you know what? If I don't have a full twenty minutes to meditate, I don't worry about it. I will take whatever I can get—even a ten-minute sit is far better than nothing.

I often think about Bob's analogy: Most of the time our mind is here, he tells every student, gesturing boldly with his arms raised in the air, hands simulating choppy waves. "What TM does is allows your mind to go deep down here," he explains, slowly lowering his arms as I visualize the calm beneath the sea. "You're still thinking, but TM is about achieving the calm that lies beneath the thunderous, crashing waves on the surface."

Bob says that the Pentagon has begun to teach meditation to soldiers suffering from post-traumatic stress, and he says it's highly effective in helping teenagers transition from high school to college, which is why Emma and Jake are considering learning some form of meditation as well. They see the calm it has brought me. As I watch the spate of race-related police incidents that have led to riots and alarmed the nation, I can't help but believe that teaching police officers meditation might greatly improve their stress levels and reduce avoidable incidents.

Within weeks of regular practice without missing a single meditation, Peter tells me that he thinks it's already had an effect on me. I push him to describe exactly what he means, and when he does I'm thrilled.

"If I had to put my finger on it," he says, "you seem more at ease."

I agree. Long after my twenty minutes are over, I notice that I can take my sense of calm out into my day and it helps me be more patient and more present. When his book came out, Dan Harris told *Men's Journal* that one of his favorite phrases had become *respond, don't react*.

"Say you're in line at Starbucks and somebody cuts you off," Dan said. "You think to yourself, 'I'm angry.' And immediately, instantaneously, reflexively, you inhabit the thought and become angry. Meditation teaches you to put a little bit of a break between the thought and the emotional state. You recognize that you're angry or annoyed or impatient, but instead of blindly going with the emotion, you have a buffer between stimulus and response. As a result, you're often the smartest person in the room. Not because of your intellectual horsepower but because of what social scientists call emotional intelligence and what I call the ability to manage your own shit."

In New York City, Uber car service has all but eclipsed the

iconic yellow taxi as a mode of transportation for many people: wherever you are, all you have to do is click on an app and a car magically appears within a few minutes. That's the easy part. The hard part, as many veteran Uber passengers will tell you, is that some drivers have no idea where they're going. Without GPS, they'd be totally lost. Even *with* GPS they're sometimes lost. There have been instances, I will admit, when I have gotten testy with these drivers. But now that I have a greater sense of awareness, I am far less likely to huff and puff with exasperation at these drivers: all that hot air isn't going to change a thing. Instead of obsessing about their questionable abilities, I simply help with directions and wish them well.

Meditation has turned me from catty to chatty.

Sometimes during my practice I experience a gap between when my exhalation stops and my inhalation starts again, which has a calming effect on me. I realize it's not so different than the phrase I adopted to help me lose weight and keep it off: *Embrace the pause.* This mini-mantra encourages me to stop, assess the situation, and decide if what I'm about to reach for is a preference (I want, I want) or a priority.

I chose TM because I know people who are longtime practitioners. But just as there are several ways to learn how to play tennis or master a foreign language, there are many other types of meditation you can explore, such as Insight Meditation, mindfulness or loving kindness meditation, and even yogic meditation. I choose to do it in the morning and evening because those times work best for my schedule. I like to sit for twenty minutes, but that might seem a bit daunting if you're just starting out. So try five minutes and then increase the time, as you're ready. I have friends who like to separate their workday from their family time by meditating for fifteen minutes or so as soon as they get home. That puts work behind them and helps them be more present for their spouse and kids. Whatever you decide, make sure your commitment is doable so that your practice continues to foster calm and relaxation, not stress and resentment.

These days, meditation instruction is everywhere: You can watch online videos, go to seminars, or check out guided imagery programs from your local library to help you find techniques to calm and quiet your mind. All of it is out there, yours for the asking.

Calm your mind, relax the effort, and embrace the pause.

Embracing the Here and Now

7

Giving acupuncture and meditation a try reminds me that we're all trying to find ways to combat stress, coping strategies to help us feel better—or at least not so lousy. For years I comforted myself with food, as many women do, but that wasn't my only source of solace. I also chose to indulge in a fantasy world of *if only*s and *I'll be happy when*s instead of committing to the hard work—physically and emotionally—of changing my relationship to my body and to my self.

In the face of life's stress and challenges, I believed that little voice inside me that assured me my unhappiness wasn't my fault. It's the same voice that millions of Powerball players hear twice a week, telling them that they needn't worry, that all their troubles will disappear *if only* their six numbers pop up on those balls. I know it's absurd to think that money alone solves life's ills. I know that tying my financial future to a random drawing with crazy odds is just dumb—I would never do that. My own *if only*s were different, I rationalized. They gave me a way to soothe the pain that comes from being trapped in a fat body, with no easy way out, and I turned to them time and again. Whenever I mention my if-only mentality to other women, they know exactly what I'm talking about. Some have their own variation on that theme. They say things like *I'll be happy when*... I lose weight... get a better job... find the perfect partner... fill in the blank.

When I was at Miami Beach Senior High School, I thought *if only* I could win the state debate championship my classmates would finally admire me and quit calling me Fat Tory. I worked my butt off—well, not literally, since the butt stayed big—and my partner and I became the first girls in Florida history to win a traditional debate trophy. The *Miami Herald* published our photos. But in my mind, nothing changed. I was still Fat Tory. When my classmate Brian called me a fat cow in history class, everyone laughed. Years later, when he heard that I recalled that awful incident in *The Shift*, he messaged me to say that he had no memory of it. But I can hear it like it was yesterday, a scar that will never disappear.

In my early twenties, I thought my career would be set *if only* I could jump from being an intern to an assistant at ABC News to a full-fledged publicist at NBC News. I did it and threw myself into the job with everything I had, working twelve-hour days, only to be fired a couple years later. That's when I decided to start my own business, which I've worked hard at to make a success, and which led to appearances on *Good Morning America* and ultimately a regular gig there.

But I was still Fat Tory.

After a lifetime of this, I think *if only* I can lose weight and be a normal-size woman, good things will come to me. And they do. I lose the weight and I keep it off. *The Shift* tops the *New York Times* bestseller list. I hear from thousands of women who identify with my story and share deeply touching stories of their own. I no longer hide from my physician. I get my first mammogram and take better care of myself. I'm a better role model for my kids. I look better and more importantly feel better, too. It's all good.

So why does my mind still race? Why do I still wake up anxious and stressed on many mornings? I worked hard. I lost the weight. I look great. I accomplished all my goals, didn't I? So why don't I hear trumpets blaring? Why don't I feel as fabulous on the inside as I do on the outside?

As I think about that, I recall that famous Smith Barney brokerage commercial from my childhood, starring actor John Houseman. It ends with him asking, "How do they make money? The old-fashioned way...they earn it." That was a profound message then and still is now. Maybe it's just me, but I think that all the shortcuts that we have at our disposal give the impression that we can fulfill all our dreams at SnapChat speed. We have come to think that getting what we want may take a bit of effort initially, but once the burst of hard work is over, we can kick back and relax.

If only we do this, we'll get that.

Want to be a famous singer? No biggie. Forget about whether you have any talent in the first place: *if only* you can just get on *American Idol* or *The X Factor*, fame and glory will come to you. Before long you'll be Taylor Swift, the girl who is now worth tens of millions of dollars, the one whose spot-on lyrics appear magically in kick-butt songs without much effort on her part. Want to gain instant stardom in anything you do? That's a breeze, too. *If only* you create a fun YouTube video, it'll go viral and the whole world will love you.

Ask anyone who has achieved fame and glory and she'll tell you that it's a lot harder than it looks. But in an era of instant gratification, with products and services designed to make our lives so much easier, that part of the equation often gets lost. Our computers are lightning fast, capable of keeping multiple tabs open at once. We're so busy multitasking that we sometimes forget the single task in front of us. The finished product that we're treated to on TV or the Web belies all the talent, training, and hard work that went into creating it. With all these time-saving gadgets and tools, we have forgotten Houseman's lesson from that iconic TV ad: Success in life takes hard work. You've got to earn it.

The truth is this mindset of *if only* and *I'll be happy when* can actually prevent us from being happy and achieving whatever joy and success mean to us. By regretting the past (*If only I hadn't let myself go…or if only I had taken that other job…I'd be so much happier*) or placing so much emphasis on the future (*I'll be happy when I lose those 20 pounds…when I find that perfect mate…when I get that promotion*) we aren't even aware of what's going on with and around us. Achieving any major life goal takes time, patience, and attention. It requires us to be present here and now, to do the work that's required to get it done. And even if we achieve that one thing—whether it's losing weight after a lifetime of obesity or becoming a famous singer or winning the lottery—there's no guarantee that it'll be the answer to our happiness prayer. There are plenty of stories of one-hit wonders in the music world and of people who won millions in the lottery and are decidedly *not* happy.

After committing to a regular meditation practice and biweekly acupuncture sessions, I've begun to rethink what happiness is all about. It's tempting to define happiness as a mental Fourth of July, with brilliant fireworks exploding into a thousand points of light. Sure, there are many moments of exhilaration in life when happiness comes in the form of the sort of mind-blowing and over-the-top experience you get at sporting events, concerts, the theater and extravagant celebrations. But I'm starting to think that real happiness and true joy are far different, perhaps somewhat less exciting in the short term but far more fulfilling over the long haul.

Happiness is a choice. It's my choice. It's your choice. It comes with a desire to embrace the totality of our experiences—the good, the bad, and the ugly—without getting stuck in the past or consumed by the future. Our attitude and our willingness to be happy are entirely within our control—among the only things that are totally up to each of us. Losing weight *was* the reward, yet my personal accomplishment wasn't nearly enough to satisfy me. Shedding all of those pounds should have been the greatest reward of all, an awesome accomplishment. Writing a heartfelt, well-received book was more than I could have ever hoped for. But I was incapable of pausing and savoring the moment and taking long-term satisfaction in it.

For many overweight women, somewhere over the rainbow is spelled T-H-I-N. I have been to the Land of Oz and, trust me, it's a swell place. But now I realize that better health is its own North Star in the night sky. I have that. I own that. It's mine. So is the bright constellation of a great family and being surrounded by people who love me. I temporarily lost sight of who and what matters.

I now realize that *if only* is a crutch that enabled me to avoid facing adversity and tackling things in my life that needed fixing. It is a convenient way out. *If only I looked that way, if only I had more money, if only I got that job…but since I didn't get that, oh well, it wasn't meant to be, and I'll just stay stuck in this lousy place.* It's a mental trick that lets me off the hook and gives me an excuse to not do the hard work, the heavy lifting that is required of all of us to use what we have to get what we want.

As I started exploring these thoughts, a friend introduced me to Oklahoma-based life coach David Leifeste. When I mentioned to him that I had grappled with this mindset throughout much of my life, he knew exactly what I was talking about and suggested that I wasn't alone.

"It's a quick fix, grass-is-greener, fountain of youth miracle mentality that precludes taking responsibility for one's life and understanding the value of a well-fought struggle and contentment verses quick-fix happiness," he said. "Immediate gratification is not where the action is for sustained success and joy."

I'm ready now to dump my *if only* security blanket once and for all and grow up. I will try to stay rooted in the here and now and show up at my life's table. That *if only* mentality was seductive and lured me into a fuzzy and complacent fantasyland, but the truth is that life comes with a series of ongoing challenges from the day we're born until the day we die. Rich or poor, young or old, fat or thin, no one is immune to adversity. That's part of the deal. The grass may seem greener on the other side but once you go there, you find that it isn't always.

Plus, better to focus on perfecting my own lawn than envying someone else's. I'd lost sight of that.

At a seminar a few weeks after my first acupuncture session, I ran into my friend Sheila, who is a bigwig in talent management and recruitment for a global company. She told me she's had a difficult week in meetings with an endless stream of people coming into her office with the same thing on their minds: they want promotions. We began to dissect the idea of being content with what you have. We talked about how to savor where you are, being good with it and getting better as opposed to always craving the next job, a more prestigious title, or wanting what "that person has." When does *now* trump *more?*

"Isn't it a sign of weakness to not crave more, to not want more?" I asked. "Shouldn't we be itching with impatience, always expecting more of ourselves, wanting to get to the next level?"

"No!" Sheila said sharply, which came as a surprise since she hasn't gotten to a senior level by being shy about what she wants. "It's okay to relish where you are and what you do and to be *really good* at it. Just because you achieve something is no reason to immediately wonder, 'Okay, what's next?' Being good with where you are right now is hardly a sign of laziness."

She's right. It's so tempting to look at life as a ladder that we must always keep climbing to be happy. We assume that the biggest prize awaits us at the top, and we forget to look sideways or even on a lower rung. The truth is that happiness can often be found at every rung, but only if we look for and embrace it. Too often from our lowly perches at work, we look at senior executives and think that life must be so sweet at the top. We fail to stop and see the bigger picture: that dealing with management problems and pressures day in and day out can be a grind, too.

It's so easy to compare ourselves to others and to envy what they have and we don't. We read about stars and think they have it all. We see the lives of friends through the lens of Facebook, where everything is oh-so-perfect, and wish we had it as good. It's a dangerous trap, yet it's so tempting.

The reality is that I already *have* a good life like so many other women do, but it took this shake-up or wakeup or whatever you want to call my fiasco funk to snap me back to reality.

After my conversation with Sheila, walking uptown along Central Park West past the Museum of Natural History, I know my whole "now that I lost weight/what's next/where's my promotion and my reward?" notion was not only wrong but has caused me unnecessary anguish and grief. It was destructive. I *have* it good—really good—but I wanted more. Oprah says it best: "If you concentrate on what you don't have, you will never, ever have enough." My *if only*s have kept me from being happy with who I am and what's going on in my life at any given moment. And yes, Oprah is right: The more I obsess about what could have, would have, or should have been (those *coulda, woulda, shoulda*s), the less satisfied I am.

My friend Laurie Dalton White is a married mother of two who runs huge women's conferences that I've spoken at in Pennsylvania, Massachusetts, and Texas. She told me that she learned this lesson in her home in Piedmont, California: In the midst of a bathroom renovation, she found herself daydreaming to the plumber. "When I win the lottery, I'll fix this and I'll do that and I'll add here," she explained pleasantly to him as she pointed to various spots that might benefit from improvements.

The man surveyed the space, looked at her, and said, "Lady, you've already won the lottery."

If you've been living an *if only* life, it may be time to recalibrate your priorities. There's a good chance you have more to be happy about than you realize. Focus more on getting joy from your everyday experiences. Be grateful for basic things: a roof over your head, food on the table, clothes on your back. If you have kids, think about their good and grounded sides, not their shortcomings. Ditto for husbands or wives or partners or friends who stick with you no matter what your body looks like or what job you have. Those intangibles matter. Who is happier, the girl who demands a four-carat engagement ring from a jerk or the girl who is grateful for a twisted pipe cleaner from a stand-up guy who thinks she hung the moon?

Commit to giving today all you've got. Then, do it again tomorrow.

8

Sleeping My Way to the Top

O kay, I admit that the title of this chapter is provocative, but I'm not referring to trading sex for a better job or more money. I really mean sleep, as in getting comfortable, closing your eyes, and moving into REM sleep.

I have been a workaholic ever since I left Emerson College in Boston after my sophomore year to find my fortune in New York. I mix life and work into a seamless entity, spending large chunks of weekends on never-ending tasks tied to my business. I choose it, embrace it, and never complain about it. I all but wear my office hours on my sleeve and I have always slept just a few hours a night, sending and responding to emails at all hours. Friends and business associates sometimes wonder what I am doing up at 3:42 a.m. on a Tuesday.

My feeling about sleep boiled down to this: *Nothing gets accomplished when I sleep, so who needs it?*

Plus, I'd read profiles of many accomplished people who

are invariably described as being so consumed by their work that they operate on little sleep, as if it's a badge of honor. They pretty much imply that sleep is overrated. As such, I infer from them that working more and sleeping less are keys to success, so I have long gone to bed late and woken up early, believing that more than five or six hours is a telltale sign of laziness. I associate a hard work ethic with minimal shut-eye.

But a talk by Arianna Huffington changes my mind entirely. In just a few minutes, she convinces me that my views on sleep are not only completely misguided but also detrimental to my health—the health that I am working so hard to regain. I know from my own experience that too little sleep can prompt me to make bad snack choices and eat larger portions. That's the story of my life: working or watching TV late at night when I should be asleep, I suddenly get the urge for tiramisu or a giant bag of potato chips and I go for one—or both. But I've never thought about the connection between lack of sleep and over-eating until I hear Arianna's talk. And when I do, I learn that cutting back on sleep increases insulin levels, which puts you at risk for Type 2 diabetes. Studies also reveal that not getting enough sleep leads to an increased risk of memory loss, bone deterioration, colon cancer, and heart disease. Sounds pretty serious to me.

Arianna knows firsthand of what she speaks.

Addressing a group of high-powered women at a TED talk in Washington, the *Huffington Post* founder says she once got by on just a few hours of sleep. Then one day she fainted from exhaustion, hit her head on her desk, and woke up in a pool of blood. She had broken her cheekbone, and a gash near her right eye required five stitches. As a result, she began to study the science of sleep, and by talking to a variety of experts learned that sleep deprivation is far more dangerous than she had ever imagined.

"I'm here to tell you, the way to a more productive, more inspired, more joyful life is getting enough sleep," she says. "We women are going to lead the way in this new revolution, this new feminist issue. We are literally going to sleep our way to the top."

The crowd roars.

No slacker herself, Arianna says that sleep deprivation has become a virility symbol among high-powered men, but that it has also infected the Type A women she is addressing. Suggest having breakfast at 8 a.m. with someone in her circle, she says, and more likely than not the response is, "That's okay—I can get in a tennis game and a few conference calls before we meet." At a dinner, she says, a man brags that he got four hours of sleep the night before. "I felt like saying, 'If you had gotten five, this dinner would be a lot more interesting.' Men think that means they are so incredibly busy and productive, but the truth is they're not."

What she says next really strikes home. Referring to the 2007 recession, she says, "We have had brilliant leaders in business, in finance, in politics, make terrible decisions. A high IQ does not mean that you're a good leader, because the essence of leadership is being able to see the iceberg before it hits the *Titanic*. We've had far too many icebergs hitting our *Titanic*s and I have a feeling that if Lehman Brothers was Lehman Brothers & Sisters, they might still be around. While the brothers were busy being hyperkinetic 24/7, maybe a sister would have noticed the iceberg because she had gotten her seven and a half or eight hours sleep and seen the big picture."

The crowd applauds. Amen to that.

Arianna recommends eight hours of sleep a night, which she says she gets ninety-five percent of the time. In an interview with CBS News, she says that making her bedroom a device-free zone went a long way toward accomplishing her goal.

"For me, the key is to take all my devices out of the bedroom and charge them in another room, because otherwise, you're going to be tempted if you wake up for whatever reason to check your texts and to check your emails, and then it's much harder to go back to sleep," Arianna says.

Ever since watching that online video of her speaking, I've made a conscious decision to go to bed earlier. While falling asleep and staying asleep aren't problems, it takes considerable effort to change my routine. I haven't yet gotten the nerve to follow Arianna's lead in making my bedroom an iPhone-free space, but I have made myself put down my phone for the night by 10 p.m., without worrying about whether or not I'll miss texts or random emails. Even though I rarely conduct serious business into the night, I still have to convince myself that nearly all communication can wait until morning.

While it takes a period of acclimation, I ultimately realize that most of the texts from friends and colleagues are frivolous chitchat at best. I also learn to stop checking and refreshing my Twitter, Instagram, and Facebook feeds and admit to myself that the photos of people and their kids or their food aren't late-night critical. I wean myself from an addictive word game on my phone, which in some ways is the hardest nighttime habit to break. The Scrabble-like game is a mini obsession and each time I fail to beat my highest score, I am compelled to go for one more round because of my crazy competitive nature. From now on, sleep is the score I choose to keep.

For years, Peter slept peacefully next to me for hours before I drifted off. With this new routine, more often than not, we shut the lights off at the same time. When I get my ideal eight hours, I generally wake up feeling well rested, which results in my having more energy and being in a better mood. I'm less likely to snap at Peter or the world. That may sound painfully obvious, but it never was to me. As Arianna says, "When everyone gets enough sleep they make better decisions, which makes for a better world."

I pull it off most nights, with the exception of Wednesdays because I wake up particularly early on Thursdays for *Good Morning America*. And sometimes getting enough sleep when I'm on the road with a packed schedule is hard. The same is probably true for anyone with a baby or a particularly grueling work schedule. Even so, getting enough sleep now becomes a priority. It joins a growing list of practices I once dismissed but now embrace.

Some experts say that your bed should be for only two activities: sex and sleeping. I won't go that far, but if you pooh-pooh the importance of sleep as I once did, I encourage you to rethink the way you prepare for bed. To get more shut-eye, work backwards: If your wake-up time has little to no wiggle room, start there and count back eight hours to determine your ideal bedtime. If possible, begin to wind down an hour or even two hours earlier. Turn off the computer, put away your phone, lower the volume on the TV (or turn it off completely), and dim the lights. Don't read or watch anything that's likely to agitate you or get your mind racing—no dire news reports or scary movies. New sheets and pillows may be a great investment if you're not already comfortable in your bed. My friend Cindy swears by spritzing lavender scent on her pillow, long thought to support better sleep. Our neighbor Stan has a small sound machine by his bed that replicates ocean and rain-forest noises that put him to sleep; he purchased it after a doctor told him that his habit of popping Ambien had to stop. We all have to figure out what works best for each of us. Check out Arianna's funny speech online. I provide a link to it at **toryjohnson.com**. Then join me in bed.

Avoid depriving yourself of sleep; it's a necessity, not a luxury.

9

Letting Go

One of the most common bits of marriage advice is "Don't go to bed angry." All you get is an uncomfortable night's sleep, which usually leads to starting the next day on the wrong foot. Seniors say that when you get old, going to bed angry can be problematic because you never know if you'll wake up or not. Better to resolve the tiff or calmly agree to continue the conversation in the morning, and say "I love you."

Although there have been exceptions over the years, Peter and I generally follow this rule. But that doesn't mean that I haven't gone to bed annoyed about all sorts of things at one time or another. Sometimes it's silly stuff, like being on the receiving end of crappy customer service when I'm trying to make an airline reservation. Or dealing with a frustrated *Good Morning America* viewer who sends a nasty tweet at 10 o'clock at night because she can't find the link to make a purchase. We all experience frustrations. But in order to continue to reduce the stress, I realize I need to work on not going to bed agitated or out of sorts.

Evening meditation is certainly far better than any pill or potion. Sometimes, though, simply sitting still isn't enough for me to let go of the events of the day and not worry about what tomorrow might bring. There are some nights when I need a way to release and surrender. So I add a layer or two to my wind-down practice by silently asking myself two questions.

The first is: What went right for me today? This allows me to think about all the things I want to celebrate—the stuff that made me smile. Some days they seem small: a funny family chat at dinner, an especially challenging workout that I completed, frizz-free hair. A lot of teeny victories make for really good days. Other nights I have bigger moments to be proud of, like an especially strong TV segment, a breakthrough with a new client, or the several hours I spent helping someone feel better about herself.

I let myself relive those smile moments, really *feel* them. I notice how my body experiences them—the tension melts away from my shoulders, my jaw releases and any knots in my neck almost magically loosen. Suddenly the not-so-great times— losing my temper or getting my feelings hurt—don't loom as large.

Of course there are nights when I notice some leftover irritation, some persistent disappointment that keeps nagging at me. So I ask myself a second question: Whom do I need to forgive? If I've allowed someone to irk me in a big or small way, I give myself permission to release my irritation. Again, sometimes the cause of my annoyance seems silly or inconsequential, like when I have a testy exchange with a cab driver or someone cuts in front of me at Starbucks. And, of course, sometimes the person I need to forgive most of all is me—for being too judg-mental or impatient with others or myself.

Leadership coach Emily Bennington tells me that she does a very similar thing. Before she goes to sleep, she asks her-self, "What do I need to let go of?" She's focused not just on people, but on all the things that may be holding her back—habits, fears, excuses. "This practice not only allows me to diffuse my brain's attachment to victim-y 'poor me' stories," Emily says, "but it also creates a sense of calm compassion that segues into deeper sleep."

It's so easy to have a zillion thoughts and fears or *whatever* swirling in your mind when you turn off the light, making it hard to let things go and setting yourself up for a toss-and-turn night. Am I good enough? Will they like me? Do I have what it takes to get what I want? Have I been kind? The same ques-tions cycle through my mind when I'm full of doubt, and they don't slow down long enough for me to answer. I have noticed one thing, however, that can help me quiet my mind enough to prevent it from getting stuck in that spin cycle. Either before getting into bed or after lying down, I tune into whatever feel-ing is the most dominant. Say I feel angry about something that happened at work. Instead of reliving all the reasons why I feel that way, and blaming all the people responsible, I acknowledge the story and simply feel whatever comes up. Where does that anger physically show up in my body? Is my jaw clamped shut? Are my fists clenched? My legs tightening? And then I see what happens when I relax my jaw, wiggle my fingers, shake out my legs, and slow down my breath. When I take the time to release the *effects* of my fears, I find that the fears themselves lose their power and it's amazing how much better I feel. Only then in the presence of calm can I focus on a sound solution. I ask myself what I can do to take control and fix what irks me. Instead of expecting someone else to figure it out, I assume responsibility and lead the way.

When something or someone is upsetting us, it's not always as easy as dropping it and moving on, though that conversation with myself is the best first step. From there, I try several other methods until I feel a sense of inner peace and true contentment.

I concentrate on my breathing. I pretend I'm breathing in and out of my heart instead of my nose. I "inhale" an image of the person I want to forgive, and I "exhale" kindness toward him or her. It takes some practice, especially if I feel particularly wounded. I might have to do it several times (especially if at first I feel like I'm only pretending to forgive) in order to let things go.

I've discovered another helpful trick to release something I believe is holding me back, which is aided by a stash of balloons I keep in a drawer. As I blow up that balloon, I imagine with every deliberate breath that I'm filling it with what I must release from inside me—the thoughts or anger that I want to let go of. I tie the balloon tightly and release it outside. Then I turn away and never look back. It's gone.

Give these "forgiveness" practices a try tonight, and then again tomorrow and the next day. After a week or so, email me at **tory@toryjohnson.com** with an update on how it's going and how you feel.

Even the most successful people must figure out how to make friends with their fears and doubts, a realization that hits home during a question-and-answer session Robin Roberts and I have at the annual Pennsylvania Conference for Women. The great Diane Keaton, the Academy Award–winning Diane Keaton, has just wowed the Philadelphia crowd, and we're up next. "Pretty good warm-up act for us," I whisper to Robin as we walk onstage to a standing ovation—it's for her, but I happily bask in Robin's glow as we take our seats.

I start by asking about Amber, Robin's partner of more than ten years. "Gee, I thought we were friends, Tory," Robin deadpans. "I expected you'd open with a softball and go from there." The audience laughs and applauds and our thirty minutes together are fun and enlightening. When our chat turns to overcoming career challenges—the fear and self-doubt that can hold us back—Robin says, "If you're going to wait for the fear to subside, you'll be sitting on the sidelines for a very long time. Just be true to yourself. Trying to be like anyone else is too hard. For me, it's easier to just be myself." The cheers are almost deafening.

She shares this advice with the sold-out crowd of eight thousand women seated in front of us, but I can't help but think she's talking directly to me.

> End each night by asking:
> What went right today?
> What am I grateful for today?
> Who must I forgive?

10

Changing Things Up

S pa Bene is a quiet mani-pedi place that has recently opened near my office. While plenty of women race in and out for a quick polish change, many opt to stay longer in the relaxing environment with soft music piping through the speakers. For me, the best thing about this place is that the owners discourage loud cell-phone conversations. Outside, the street is a cacophonous truck route, but none of that seems to permeate the atmosphere inside.

I'm meeting Jill Donovan here. She owns Rustic Cuff, an Oklahoma-based jewelry company that specializes in—you guessed it—cuffs. I have featured her cuffs on "Deals & Steals" a few times and the line is always a big hit with viewers. It's cool outside but Jill shows up wearing black cotton shorts and ankle boots, revealing tan, toned legs. I'm not sure why she even bothered with the coat and gloves; I'd be flaunting those legs if mine looked like hers. She wears her blond hair in a short, sharply cropped cut that makes her look a little like Suze Orman. Why not combine a little pleasure with business, we both agree, as we relax in our leather pedicure chairs.

Until now, she has always pitched products to me by email and mail. This time she gets to see my reaction in person. She unwraps several samples of leather cuffs that she's designed. I tell her that if she's able to get the prices down by a few dollars per piece and manufacture them in bright colors—not just black—they'd be a hit with my viewers and would look great on TV.

Leaving the office at midday for any reason is a new thing for me. For years I'd invariably order in lunch and eat at my desk. I worried about losing productivity or missing out on something oh-so-important. I was terrified that all hell would break loose if I dared break away. On top of it, I had convinced myself that I was far too busy to step out. So busy that I couldn't even spare fifteen or twenty minutes, let alone an hour, away from my office.

The truth is that *busy* and *successful* are not synonymous, as I've told countless audiences. The same is true for *busy*, *successful*, and *happy*. So I've begun to rethink my work habits. I started reading up on the research that demonstrates the benefits of short breaks during work, to stretch, take a walk, eat, catch up with coworkers, or even get your toes done. Several studies even suggest that letting your mind wander boosts your creativity and problem-solving abilities. I'm game for that, which is why I now make a point to get out of the office at lunchtime, if not every day, then most days. Sometimes I walk around the block a couple of times, or venture farther afield, especially when the weather cooperates. Other days I find an errand to do in the neighborhood or meet Peter for a quick bite at the little sushi place next door that caters to the lunch-in-a-hurry crowd. Just the slightest break from work can make all the difference in my day. I return refreshed, ready to tackle the afternoon without falling into that typically tiring 3 p.m. slump.

The biggest discovery has come from doing things that I once took for granted, as well as things that were outside my comfort zone. Thanks to my new routine, I've headed out a few times at noon to the main branch of the New York Public Library, an iconic building that I hadn't set foot in for more than twenty years, even though it's not too far from my office. During lunch one day, I spend a half hour taking in the grandeur of its famous reading room, simply watching students and scholars working at the long rows of lamp-lit tables. On another visit, I spend a few minutes people-watching at the foot of Patience, one of the marble lions (along with Fortitude) that guard the steps in front of this grand building. The lions remind me of the patience I have gained since making small changes in my life and the fortitude with which I have committed to maintaining them.

Another day I walk across Central Park and spend an hour taking in a fabulous exhibit of twentieth-century artists like Jackson Pollock and Edward Hopper at the Metropolitan Museum of Art. It is just a taste, but I love the feeling of being a tourist in my own city. I've deliberately taken different routes for short walks just to switch things up a little each week.

I even dared once to take the abbreviated one-and-a-half-hour Circle Line cruise around Manhattan and listened as the tour guide pointed out things about the city that I never knew before. Far more significant than that is that I did this alone, something that I never have done much of before. There's a unique satisfaction in going it alone. It's not better or worse than sharing the experience with someone else, just different. With the Hudson River two blocks to the west, I sometimes walk there and stare at it. There's something very soothing, even therapeutic about walking near water, whether it's the beach in Miami or the reservoir in Central Park. Just gazing at water for as little as ten minutes resets my mood.

Writers have long talked about the soothing effects of water. Henry David Thoreau said a lake is "Earth's eye, looking into which the beholder measures the depth of his own nature." Author Annie Dillard said that the sea "pronounces something, over and over, in a hoarse whisper; I cannot quite make it out." And novelist Joseph Conrad once wrote, "The true peace of God begins at any spot a thousand miles from the nearest land."

Since I've begun to get out more, I've yet to return to work to discover that the sky has fallen or that business has tanked in my absence. While the women in my office prefer to bring their lunch to eat at their desks, I encourage them to leave early to soak up the weather, to enjoy some free time, to avoid a hectic commute. Sometimes it's not the boss who tells us we can't leave our desks, it's our own inner voice that convinces us we can't step away and that if we do it means we're slacking off. I can't ever remember hearing any eulogy that praised the deceased for the number of hours they sat at their desks.

I subscribe to the Facebook page of *Humans of New York*, a daily stream of photographs of people in the city and their pointed thoughts. One of my favorite posts is a 2011 photo of a ninety-three-year-old woman named Mary, pictured sitting on a ledge outside a building. "If you force yourself to go outside, something wonderful always happens," she says. Many fans of the page commented that they were adopting that as their new life motto. I'm among them.

If you're stuck in a routine that keeps you at your desk, whether it's at home or in an office, look for ways to break it up. Get up and walk around your neighborhood or corporate park or wherever your day finds you. It's a bonus if there's an ocean, lake, or river nearby, but I've found that simply looking at a fountain or pool for a few minutes works, too. Like meditation and exercise, changing your environment is another tool in your Shift kit.

Changing one thing in your life can give you the power to change anything.

TAKING CARE OF BUSINESS

The only way to do great work is to love what you do. If you haven't found it yet, keep looking. Don't settle.

—*Steve Jobs*

Make Hard Decisions Gracefully

11

When I was twenty-two and the publicist at NBC's *Dateline*, a new boss came in and fired our entire PR department. I loved my job, excelled at it, and was desperate to stay at NBC News. But none of that mattered when I went to his office and begged him to keep me. He leaned back in his big leather chair, hands behind his head, and said coldly, "Tory, it's a big world out there and I suggest you go explore it." For weeks I explored nothing but pints—plural—of Haagen Dazs.

Ultimately I had a choice: I could stay depressed and do nothing and continue to watch my bank account dwindle, or I could snap out of it. That's when I made my very first life shift, although at the time I didn't recognize it as such. As a result of that searing experience, I decided I never wanted to be in a position where one person, one project, or one paycheck would derail me. My career had hit a rock, but I knew other women were just starting to explore theirs and needed help, so I had an idea: Job fairs were a dime a dozen, but I'd never heard of one specifically geared to women. Why not help them find the jobs they're so qualified to do?

Women For Hire, my women's career expo company, was born, followed a few years later by Spark & Hustle, a conference series designed to teach women entrepreneurs how to turn their passion into profit. Helping women make it happen became my life's focus. And it still is. I connect thousands of smart and savvy women with top employers. I give women small-business owners the tools and resources they need to thrive on their own. My overriding message is to tap what you have to get what you want and never give up.

Business was great and so, in 2007, when Peter decided to take the buyout package from *USA Today*, it made perfect sense for him to join my business. He had been a reporter and a writer his entire career and wasn't the least bit interested in managing staff or making the big decisions. "I'll help you as much as I can, but I hope you're not counting on me to generate money," he said a few days before he kissed the newspaper world good-bye after three decades. "I'm just the help; you're the rainmaker. Are you cool with that?"

"You can lean on me," I told him. "I'll handle the money stuff."

Neither of us gave much thought to what he'd actually *do* around the office, figuring it would just work itself out. And to a large extent it did. I was happy to be working together; Peter is easy to have around and helps me with a wide range of projects. His antics make my staff guffaw, just as they did in the *USA Today* newsroom.

His intellect and sense of humor are what initially attracted me to him in the early 1990s. As the publicist at *Dateline*, it was my job to convince reporters to write stories about the newsmagazine. Since Peter wrote a high-profile column, my priority was to get to know him. The lifting was easy because he's quick and funny. He teased me relentlessly and during long phone conversations—with him at *USA Today*'s office in Rosslyn, Virginia, and me at 30 Rock in New York—we soon had an easy rapport. Conversations quickly veered away from *Dateline* into personal stuff.

He was in his late thirties with two young children and, as I soon learned, his marriage was unraveling. Although we met a few times in New York and at a TV conference in California, we primarily conducted our friendship long-distance. We talked several times a day (pre-email, of course), but I was still stunned the day he told me he loved me. Initially I thought he must be putting me on. *He's so "normal-looking," why would someone like him want a fat girl like me?* We married a year later, surrounded by family and friends at a restaurant in Tribeca, with Peter's son, Nick, then eight, as his best man. Peter relocated to New York, the center of the media industry, and continued writing his column right up until the end of his time at *USA Today*.

Without his salary, supporting our family suddenly became my responsibility and mine alone. I had to run the office and keep close tabs on revenue and expenses, mainly by hosting dozens of events each year. I do all of that in addition to my work for *Good Morning America*. Peter still marvels at my ability to push my business agenda with staffers and teasingly calls me The Hammer. He is more than happy to not have to manage anyone at work because he never had to and never wanted to in his career. He's much happier managing Marly's need to go for a walk every few hours.

Everything hummed along nicely until after *The Shift* came out, when I began to lose interest in the very businesses I had worked so hard to build. The offer for a new TV gig that I was expecting to come through went from sure thing to no-thing and several loyal employees jumped ship. All my post-*Shift* doldrums created a crisis of confidence in me and caused me to second-guess my normally spot-on business acumen. Suddenly I felt overwhelmed. Instead of feeling grateful for Peter's help, I resented him for his lack of a paycheck and began to take all my frustrations, fears of failing, and disappointments out on him. For such a smart, creative guy, I thought, why can't he make money? Why can't he contribute more to the bottom line?

Of course Peter didn't deserve any of this. Plus, with thousands of unemployed journalists out there, most of whom are at least half his age, asking him to go back to "a real job" was impractical at best.

On my good days, I saw definite upsides to Peter being a part of my business. Not being tied to another employer meant we could travel together, and he could handle many parenting and family obligations with ease. That flexibility counted for a lot. He could be available to take his ninety-two-year-old dad to appointments, and he could fly to Miami when he needed to help my mom now that she's alone. When he's not busy with those big-ticket items, he's covering so much of the day-to-day. I never even have to think about grocery shopping, changing the oil in our car, or a zillion other things that keep our home and family running smoothly. How can I find fault with a man who is so thoughtful that he removes the stems and washes strawberries before placing them in a bowl in our refrigerator? He does all of the stuff that nobody else thinks about.

But still, I continued to pick at him.

"I don't need a helper," I tell him bitterly after seeing revenue dip one quarter. "I need an earner."

"That's not the deal we made going into this," he snaps back. "And now you want to change the rules?"

"It's not fair to dump it all on me," I say, angry and annoyed.

"Yup, and it's not fair to lay your problems at my feet," he shoots back.

"Who said life was fair?" I ask, giving him a taste of one of his favorite lines.

Variations of this spat go on for months. No one walks out or throws glasses across the room, and nothing of consequence happens as a result. But I look for reasons to pick at him and his resentment toward me grows day by day. We move on after each encounter, but I still don't like what's happening and I really don't like how I'm acting. And yet I can't quite help myself. What especially troubles me is that while some couples fight about money all the time, Peter and I have always been on the same exact page about it. I've never hidden a purchase from him, the way many of my girlfriends do with their spouses, and we've never argued about a bill or an expense. Although we have always been in sync about all money matters, and yet my own worries and insecurities about money have caused me to take my anxieties out on him.

Looking back, none of my actions made much sense—he hadn't changed and he certainly didn't create my mess—but I felt backed into a corner and I used the person closest to me as a punching bag. I was moody and bitchy; I snapped more than once that he should think about getting a job, that it was unfair to put all the pressure on me. The truth was, of course, that I didn't want him to get another job; I loved having him right where he was—with me. But under siege, we often say and do things that we don't really mean and sometimes it takes its toll. At least that was true for me. Things finally settled down and the snapping and bitchiness subsided in favor of getting the work done. Not one to hold a grudge, Peter put those incidents behind us. But I came to realize that my actions had been rude and unnecessary; they were reflections on me, not him, and I was wrong to make him the brunt of my frustrations and fears. But I didn't apologize to him for a long time—not until after I started changing my own behavior through better self-care.

And then, on a trip home from Los Angeles months later, during a random conversation with him, I find myself apologizing. I have just completed my first and only live cooking segment of *Shift* recipes on *The Talk*, the daytime show on CBS. Peter is ribbing me about how fun it was for him to watch on a monitor backstage as I guided hosts Julie Chen and Sheryl Underwood on chopping and mixing ingredients to prepare cauliflower fried "rice"—subbing cauliflower for the rice so it's a fraction of the carbs of the real deal. That's because Peter is the chef in our family. He handles every bit of meal planning, and even does the dishes. So we both find it a bit comical that I'm leading a cooking segment. "Thank goodness the dress rehearsal wasn't televised," he says, rolling his eyes. "Let's keep it between us that you had trouble identifying a measuring cup."

I'm on a high from the segment—reading emails from friends and tweets from strangers who watched—and I feel closer to

Peter than ever. Suddenly I turn to him and say, "I'm sorry I made my mess your mess."

"What do you mean?" he asks. He is clearly puzzled since my apology is out of the blue and feels like a non sequitur to him.

"You didn't sign up to be the answer to my woes," I say as I explain my better-late-than-never mea culpa.

As I think more about what drove me to such negativity, I realize that I failed to honor our agreement, which was that I'd handle the money end. I had every right to change my mind, of course, but it wasn't fair to Peter for me to be snippy without sharing what was really behind my agitation. I should have worked through that difficult time *with* Peter, instead of secretly resenting him for not intuiting why I was in such a funk in the first place. My apology—those all-important words "I am sorry"—allows me to put the whole ugly period behind me and I promise Peter (and myself) that I'll do better from now on. I know now that when I'm feeling pressure, I must be more honest and forthright with Peter and others. It's the right thing to do and would have made him feel better and more connected to what I was doing, and I would have felt much less overwhelmed, too.

While I'm focused on digging into work, Peter and the kids begin looking at colleges. I'm having a lot of trouble wrapping my head around the fact that both Emma and Jake will be leaving home in the fall, but I'm eager to hear how things are going. From the reports I get via text, email, and phone, they're having a blast. They've seen a variety of schools including Syracuse University, Peter's alma mater. Emma regales me with a story of how their student guide boasted about having a dual major in journalism and English. Peter, who graduated with that same major in 1976, says under his breath, "Good luck with that, bud." Jake grabs the phone from her and tells me about how Peter dragged them away from the tour to show exactly where he sat in an amphitheater for a psychology class forty years ago. "When the Bee Gees were popular and John Travolta had a thirty-inch waist," Emma quips in the background, mimicking her dad. "Stayin' alive," I hear Peter say.

The three of them also tour the University of Maryland and Johns Hopkins. Jake returns from Baltimore loving Hopkins, especially the robotic surgical lab. He notes that the benches that dot the campus are identical to the ones in Central Park, his backyard a block from our apartment. Emma is impressed with the big school pride at Maryland, but worries that with a low out-of-state acceptance rate, she won't get in. She settles for a selfie with a bronze terrapin, the school mascot.

I join them one weekend to see a handful of universities in Boston, and within a few hours both kids seem to be bitten by the Beantown bug. They've heard me tell stories about my two years at Emerson and Peter talks endlessly about summers as a kid on Cape Cod, just a few hours away. Plus, everyone knows that Boston is the quintessential college town.

While we don't push it, Peter and I secretly hope that the kids will attend colleges in the same town. While it would obviously save us from making separate drop-offs, pick-ups, and visits, more important is that they'd be near each other. When you're twins who love and like each other and would do anything to help one another out, proximity is important. Our family knows this without talking about it.

I have friends who have been saving for their daughters' weddings since they were little girls. But giving Emma a princess moment at the altar has never been my fantasy. Peter and I want to give both Emma and Jake a strong financial launch by letting them graduate without student debt. My parents paid my way for two years at Emerson until I dropped out, and Peter's parents paid for a full ride at Syracuse.

That's what we're going to do. We've decided to skip the pricey summer vacation so we can save more for college. We keep our decision to ourselves because the kids don't need to know everything about our finances. But we're relieved that they don't want to return to sleep-away camp for the summer or take a big trip as they've done in the past. They joined their school classmates on a Holocaust trip to Poland and Germany during spring break, so for now their wanderlust seems to be sated.

Jake will still go to Brown University for a summer biomed lab program: Science is his passion and he's been looking forward to the course all year. An accident in his public high school's chemistry class severely burned a student, which led to a shutdown of all lab work on school premises. My boy was reduced to learning science by watching YouTube videos. Emma plans to devote her summer to building a budding bracelet business that she has conceived. She's made some tentative inroads selling online and developing a following and is eager to see what she can accomplish when school days and homework don't interfere with her business.

Our whole family has learned some valuable lessons these last few years. Peter and I struggled through financial and personal challenges as we moved from having two incomes to relying on my salary alone. Emma and Jake are making bigger decisions that will impact their futures. My takeaway? When the going gets tough or you're feeling under siege, don't turn on the people closest to you. Accept that hard decisions are inevitable and own them, even when they're not particularly fun or popular, or when backing down might seem easier in the moment but unwise in the long run.

Be willing to own your mistakes along with your successes.

Work at Work

12

My determination to Shift for Good has pulled me back from my emotional abyss and helped me recommit my strengths and focus on the present. All of this newfound calm and connectivity comes not a moment too soon.

My businesses needed me. When my post-*Shift* euphoria, followed by numbing depression, consumed me, I pretty much checked out of my day-to-day responsibilities. I watched blankly as three staffers walked out the door over a remarkably short period of time. One had been with me since 1999, when I founded Women For Hire. When a second saleswoman left shortly after *The Shift* was published, I rationalized that young women change jobs a lot these days. Even when my right hand at Spark & Hustle quit, instead of sensing danger, I told myself that she needed a new challenge.

"Maybe you should have made some attempt, any attempt, to keep her," Peter suggested when I told him what had happened.

"I don't want someone working for me who doesn't want to

89

be here," I huffed, a not-so-subtle hint that I didn't want to discuss it.

"Maybe she just wanted to talk," he continued, trying to engage me, but he knew the conversation was over. What was done was done.

Of course now I realize I blew it. As someone who advises other women on small business, I violated a golden rule: Value the folks who row for you and keep them happy and engaged. Instead of acting like the boss, I acted like a child when my trusted aide told me she was unhappy. I didn't even express my disappointment that she was moving on or my gratitude for all she had done.

In a moment of raw, honest self-reflection, I realize now that it was my fault these staffers left. They could tell that I had checked out. I had been off in my own little world. I had ignored their progress and taken longer than usual to respond to their questions and concerns. Peter had warned me that I needed to pay more attention, but I brushed him off by claiming, "I'm *always* available." Yet that was disingenuous: I wasn't, not really. It might not have been such a big deal in a large office where employees have multiple supervisors, but in a small operation face time with the boss matters. I failed them and I failed myself. This mess was my doing, and mine alone to fix.

If I am going to Shift for Good, I tell myself, I will have to focus on all aspects of my life. I already have the weight-loss thing down, my health is better than it's been in years, and now I need to concentrate on getting my business self back on track. And that's what I do. I stop coasting and checking out and vow to re-engage in my work, using three simple, straightforward steps.

First, I restructure my business by ramping up my private consulting and de-emphasizing big events with high overhead costs. Second, I partner with people who complement my strengths instead of replacing full-time employees, which saves me money. Joining forces with my friend Jenn Lee, an Orlando-based business coach, quickly leads to landing a few new clients: an accountant who wants to secure endorsement deals from software companies, a nutritionist who has just received her certification and needs help setting up shop, and an aesthetician eager to generate media coverage for her spa's services. And third, I decide to make money the old-fashioned way: I dial for dollars myself, instead of expecting others to generate revenue for me.

I also create a Top 50 list of prospects I believe would benefit from working with me. One by one I reach out to each one on that list. When they respond, I remove them from the tally and add other prospects so that I always have an active list. I also return to a ritual called "five by five," connecting directly with five people every day by 5 p.m. Emails and voice-mail messages don't count if they go unanswered. I push myself to make five meaningful live connections each business day.

Sticking to these basics, I begin to see results. Some people tell me they're surprised that I'm reaching out: they didn't know I offered private consulting. Others say that my fees are a lot more reasonable than they expected. And some people say no, which I expected. If I never hear "no," there's very little chance of getting a "yes" because it means I'm not reaching out to enough people.

During my crazy clouded funk, I figured that if someone wanted to work with me, they'd call. I certainly made it easy enough for people to find me—I use every major form of social media, not to mention email and phone. But looking back, that was just an excuse to prevent me from doing the hard work, the proactive effort, myself.

Another change I make is to return to my regular get-togethers with Dora, my accountant. For years I met with her every month without fail, to stay abreast of our finances. I didn't want surprises, and knowing where my business stood at all times was both essential and empowering. For fifteen years I never missed a powwow. But then I began to make excuses about not being available. I had the time but I just didn't want to hear bad news, so I avoided those meetings. It was akin to allowing mail to pile up unopened: if you don't actually lay eyes on the bills, the overdue balance might magically disappear, right? *If only!*

But now with my head in the game, and looking forward and not back, I'm ready for whatever she tells me. I hired Dora as a bookkeeper during Women For Hire's infancy when I leased office space above a Domino's Pizza in a small building on the Upper West Side. My friend Genevieve proposed the name for my company. "It'll be provocative," she said, and I agreed. A neon red WOMEN FOR HIRE sign hung on our front window overlooking a busy street. Every week or so, men would call to ask if they could hire a woman. No, no, we said, this is not *that* kind of place. We added .COM to the neon sign and the calls stopped immediately: the creeps looked it up before dialing.

At the time, Dora was about to graduate from New York University. She is wise beyond her years, having grown up in a family-run business. She's a street-smart, subway-riding New York City kid who never hesitates to deliver the truth, backed up by hard facts. She left me a few years later to join an accounting firm but continues to handle my books and now, as a CPA, our taxes. I have absolute trust in Dora, and Peter adores her. If anything ever happened to Peter and me, Dora would handle the money for the kids. That's how much we trust her.

Now, perhaps sensing that I anticipate bad financial news, Dora immediately puts me at ease by saying that losing the three employees actually helped my bottom line because we are no longer paying their salaries. With a few other recent cutbacks that I don't even feel, like downgrading services that we rarely use, we have saved even more. She's impressed with the new clients I have recently secured for my expanded consulting services and buoyed even more when I tell her I've just signed others. We agree that my renewed commitment to staying on top of things is putting us back to exactly where we want to be businesswise.

"The news is a lot better than I thought," I say to Peter after returning from our coffee date down the street. "It's actually not bad at all."

"I'm stunned," he says. "You sure she wasn't just being nice?"

"You know Dora," I say. "She has no trouble being the heavy."

The next day, after my *Good Morning America* segment, I meet Barbara Corcoran, the well-known realtor and *Shark Tank* star. We first met years ago in the green room at *Good Morning America* before going on the air and immediately hit it off. We're friends—not the kind of pals who hang out regularly, but we text every so often and get together at least once a year for a long chat.

Champignon Cafe, a few blocks from her Upper East Side

apartment and office, is a decidedly casual but reliable spot. Barbara, dressed in fitted white jeans, a navy top, and bright neon-yellow Converse sneakers, feels comfortable enough there to skip wearing any makeup for breakfast. We sit at a window table that she reserves just minutes before I arrive. A former waitress, Barbara insists I stay seated while she gets up and orders scrambled eggs for me and a toasted bagel for herself. She returns with two paper plates, iced coffee, and juice. There is no small talk. We dive right into a conversation, which I see as a mark of mutual respect. She begins to pump me with questions about my businesses, *Good Morning America*, and my life.

I confide to her that I had been in a personal and professional funk, but have taken concrete steps to come out of it. I tell her that a string of disappointments hit me hard, real hard. "I was surprised by how much it impacted me. It definitely didn't just roll off my back," I say. I brace for her to chastise me for admitting a weakness, as opposed to putting on a strong face. Instead, she says that she understands completely.

"Of *course* it hurt you," she says. "But it all comes down to how well you take a hit and how long you take to feel sorry for yourself," she says. "My advice: Get up quickly and play up what you've got."

It's so easy to become lulled into complacency, especially when no drill sergeant is telling you what to do. Most of the time no one is watching and it's up to each of us to monitor ourselves. Sometimes checking out is willful: We knew we were tired behind the wheel of the car because we were yawning. But we ignored the warning sign and tried to tough it out and the next thing we knew, our car had crashed. Other times it's passive: We simply turn a blind eye to whatever problems we face. It's easier to ignore them than to roll up our sleeves, get dirty, and fix what's wrong.

From my own business's near collapse, I learned the hard way that I can't check out; I need to pay attention every single day to clues that indicate trouble, and then deal with whatever is going on in real time, as vexing and headache-inducing as that might be.

If you slip in your personal or professional life, don't abandon hope. Get back up quickly and recommit. That's what I do to this day. When I fall off the food wagon and eat things that I know are no-no's, I get moving again immediately—before my eating gets the better of me. After two weeks of no change on the scale—morning weigh-ins have been part of my daily accountability for three years—I've finally lost a pound. A teeny victory that might be attributed to cutting down on iced coffee, which I drink with cream. Shaking things up will often move the needle. I refuse to give in to complacency and return to my old ways. I won't allow a bad meal to turn into a bad week—or more. Day One can be at any moment. That was a big lesson I learned during my Shift. It has served me well in all aspects of my life and I hope it will do the same for you. Act decisively and without regret. Own your decisions and commitments and treat yourself as though you are your own best friend at work and at home.

Make today your Day One.

LIFE KEEPS HAPPENING

You learn to rise above a lot of bad things that
happen in your life. And you have to keep going.

—*Lauren Bacall*

13

Mind the Money

S ometimes it takes a crisis to wake us up and make us pay attention to the details of our daily lives that we have long ignored. This happened to our family as my father lay dying from pancreatic cancer.

The stunned look on my mom's face just days before he died is forever etched in my mind. As news from the hospital became grim, we asked his longtime partner, Jose, to meet with us to make sure things in their architectural practice were in order.

My parents' modest ranch house is a few blocks from the Atlantic Ocean, just north of classic Miami Beach beachfront hotels like the Fontainebleau and the Eden Roc. David and I grew up there, on a small, upper-middle-class island featuring homes that were built around a public golf course in the late 1940s and early '50s. In recent years the neighborhood has gentrified, with new-money people gutting homes or razing them to build sleek McMansions on small, sixty-by-one-hundred-twenty-foot lots. But my parents' house looks roughly the same as it did in 1990, when they added a lap pool and lush tropical

landscaping, which kept my father busy most weekends pruning and trimming.

In the three weeks since he was diagnosed, it has been a
whirlwind of activity. There have been appointments with the
leading specialists in Miami, research, and family time. But
now as the prognosis becomes more dire, it's time to get an
answer to something that has been worrying my mom.

I haven't seen Jose for quite a while. He and my dad have
been partners for twenty years, which amazes some people who
know my dad since he is a difficult man: impatient, demanding,
mercurial, moody, and exacting. But as far as anyone can tell,
the two have never argued. A balding Miami Beach Jew and a
Cuban-born Catholic with jet-black hair and a limp from childhood polio, they like each other personally and professionally.
An unlikely partnership based on mutual respect, it's worked
very well for both of them. I had envisioned someday sitting
across from Jose, now in his late forties, and having this talk,
but certainly not now.

After some initial pleasantries, I ask him about the key man
policy—insurance coverage on a business partner's life in case
one "key man" dies. Such policies are intended to ensure the
business continues and each partner's family is taken care of.

"What policy?" Jose asks, momentarily startled as he shakes
his head. "We talked about it years ago but we never got around
to it." He's not contentious, just stating a fact, just like my dad
would do. My mom's eyes instantly register a combination of
shock and pain. Jose seems equally stunned by her reaction.

My mom hadn't misunderstood anything: my father led her
to believe years ago that a key man was a done deal. But as Jose
says, they "never got around to it." *And no one ever got around*

to telling her. With her husband in grave condition in intensive care, the pain of betrayal on her face is palpable. She is devastated.

The next few days are a blur. I return to New York and try to keep my mind on my work between calls to doctors and listening to my mom's optimistic but misguided certainty that my dad will recover. In the middle of all this, I'm counting the days until I become an aunt again.

David and his wife, Julie, are already the parents of Charlotte, my winsome eighteen-month-old niece. Two days after I get back home, Julie gives birth to a healthy nine-pound boy they name Morgan. My mom and the nurses manage to awaken my dad with the news and he cracks a smile for the first and only time since his condition began to deteriorate. My mom reads his reaction as a hopeful sign because, as she always says, babies bring good luck. Maybe Morgan's arrival signals a turnaround.

But a few days later his condition worsens and his internist calls David and me to alert us. We immediately fly to Miami. Late that night, my dad is gone.

At the memorial service the next week, Emma and Jake remember their grandfather as funny and fun to be with, generous with his time and money. They have always had a special bond with him that no one else in the family can claim. No one else, period. They "get" one another and always have. As early as elementary school, their relationship was defined by the emails and text jokes that flew between Miami Beach and New York.

The biggest smiles come when they share the memory of him asking them this question straight-faced when they were both in second grade.

"What begins with 'F' and ends in 'U-C-K?'"

"We couldn't believe he was asking us such a thing since we were only seven," Emma says.

"Until he gave us the answer, which was FIRETRUCK," Jake says as everyone erupts into laughter.

Standing together, David and I describe an imperfect father but talented architect with a quirky sense of humor who was devoted to the city he loved. A front-page obituary in the *Miami Herald* describes Les Beilinson as a visionary preservationist who saved large sections of Miami Beach from the bulldozers. He was the leading force behind the revival of hotels and restaurants in the famed Art Deco district on South Beach. The list of his design accomplishments is long and includes the Delano and a slew of other notable hotels, the Lincoln Road Mall, and the neon-lit arch supporting a football that graced Ocean Drive for the 2010 Super Bowl. At any given time, he had a dozen or so projects in the works: hip storefronts, trendy restaurants, hotel restorations, and new condo high-rises. I tell the congregation that had it not been for our mom, Sherry, it might never have occurred to him to venture outside Miami Beach even for a few days. She's the one who opened his eyes to travel and who was there for him every step of the way.

From the pulpit, I see middle-aged women clutching the arms of their husbands, many of them my dad's age. Soldiers talk about finding God in foxholes, but something along those lines happens at funerals, too. Funerals remind us that life is fleeting and that death can come at any time. They reignite our appreciation for the people closest to us, so much so that it prompts us to literally hang on to them. I'm not about to reveal to the congregation what we know about the insurance money.

To what end? But seeing my mom's anguished face tempts me to tell the women there, "Go home and talk about finances. Today. Right now. Don't experience the headache and heartache of finding out you've been hosed when it's too late to do anything about it."

But of course I don't.

My mom tells me later that two close friends she confided in had those very conversations with their husbands, and they've subsequently taken steps to get their affairs in order. It's the least she can do for her girlfriends. Months later, I tell a group of New York Life agents in Manhattan that their mission is to give clients the tools they need to plan for the unexpected. "Women avoid uncomfortable conversations," I say. "I didn't want to talk about my weight my whole life and I paid the price by living in a body I disliked." I tell them that my mom avoided grilling my father on estate planning because it felt awkward and unseemly, especially since she assumed it was a done deal. Then he died and she was stunned to learn that her assumptions were wrong. There was no life insurance. "We bury our heads at the prospect of discussing unpleasant subjects," I say as the women life insurance agents nod in mutual understanding. "It's your job to prevent your clients from doing that. Force them to talk. Force them to plan properly."

My mom trusted my dad, believing that because his paycheck showed up every two weeks she was set. Based on that steady salary and all his high-profile projects, she assumed he had his affairs in order. In fact, she expected it. He had been, after all, the sole breadwinner for the past twenty-five years. As such, they lived large for more than two decades. Setting aside target retirement funds was something on a to-do list that never became a priority because both of them expected him to work indefinitely, and no one expected him to die so young.

Unbelievably, just seven months earlier, my father also had allowed a six-figure term life insurance policy to lapse—one he had held for thirty years. In emails we find later, he complains about it costing him too much; a longtime broker friend promises to find more affordable alternatives. Then neither of them does anything about it, unbeknownst to my mom. We find a cancelation letter buried in a pile of opened mail on his desk. This means that not one but *two* life insurance policies my mom thought were in effect do not exist. It's the ultimate indignity for this loyal, sixty-four-year-old, stay-at-home wife who married my dad when she was all of twenty-one and he was twenty-two. How do you grieve the sudden loss of your husband of forty-three years after you discover that he has left you in a financial lurch?

Our concern about her finances threatens to overshadow our shock and grief over his sudden death, which is jarring and unnerving for all of us. It's a giant mess that no one knows about except our immediate family. It makes accepting heartfelt condolences from friends somewhat problematic because a side of us is seething: *If you only knew.*

It wasn't until I left for college in 1988 that my father's business skyrocketed, when South Beach began to morph into the world-class tourist spot it is today. Throughout my childhood, my mom worked six days a week at a children's clothing store her uncle owned. She hired, fired, and managed staff. She kept track of inventory to maximize sales to picky moms. She even escorted out junkies who wandered into the store. On her feet from morning to night, she came home exhausted. I'd tag along

Shift for Good   105

on Saturdays, and my most vivid memory is of her picking up clothes from the dressing room floor and rehanging them. Having watched her do this thousands of times, I never leave clothing in a dressing room and I've taught Emma never to do it, either: no saleswoman should have to bend over to clean up our mess.

In those years, my dad worked long hours building his fledging architecture practice. Subsidized by my mom's income, he accepted low pay in order to amass a portfolio of projects that would prove him worthy of bigger, more lucrative gigs. Later, in the 1980s, my mom opened an antiques shop on South Beach that attracted designers as the area began to gentrify. The shop quickly flourished, and on weekends my dad repaired and refinished Art Deco clocks, lamps, and furniture they bought at estate sales and flea markets. He'd marvel as my mom doubled, tripled, and quadrupled their investment. It was the happiest time in their marriage.

But she hasn't worked since closing Metropolis Flamboyant Furnishings in the early 1990s to care for my grandfather, my dad's dad, after he had a stroke. For months she fed him and helped him dress and bathe until he got back on his feet. No one needed to ask her to care for her father-in-law. It's just the way she is. Plus, she didn't need to work: my dad's six-figure income not only supported them but paid for trips to Europe and South America. This time, the antiques they brought home were for themselves, not for resale. His income also covered annual over-the-top birthday parties for Emma and Jake and now Charlotte. As doting grandparents they insisted on paying for them even though none of us asked for or expected it. Like a well-oiled machine that never ran out of steam, they also

backed David in his work producing independent documentary films, a field where filmmakers are always scrambling for
funds.

Now there is no chance my mom will go out and get a job,
and no one expects her to. She has no interest in working, but
even if she did her chances of getting hired are slim to none. I
have built a business around women and careers, and I follow
the hiring scene much like a stockbroker eyes the Dow. I have
watched the job market tumble since the recession. I know that
my aging mom, who hasn't held a job in years, is hardly desir-
able. That's not to say that she lacks talent and ability. On the
contrary, for a decade she managed dozens of my Women For
Hire career expos across the country. It's a role that involves
making sure that key aspects come together: setting up pipe
and drape backdrops, tables, and chairs; collating handouts;
arranging snacks, lunch, and giveaways; managing temporary
help and keeping my clients happy. A natural-born event plan-
ner, my mom was the glue that bound all the different parts.
She excelled at her duties, sweating each detail and doing whatever it took to make every event a success for employers and
job seekers alike. She made me look like a career expo goddess
every time.

So, while my mom is smart, skilled, and capable, none of
that transfers easily in our youth-obsessed job market. As far
as employment is concerned, she is done. And in light of all that
has transpired, she risks outliving her savings without any ability to generate new income. At the very least, she will be forced
to sharply reduce her spending and downgrade her lifestyle.
The mom who has always been there for my brother and me,

emotionally as well as financially, is about to be forced to sell her home of forty years.

I know, her situation is hardly dire and a lot of people in this world have it much worse. But she's my mom. I love her and I want her to have every joy in her golden years. After supporting my father as he built his practice and then caring for our family for all those years, she deserves to have the peace of mind that financial security brings. It breaks my heart, but there's only so much I can do besides love her and support her all I can. Unfortunately, what's done is done and we all need to move forward, in a way no one ever expected.

My mother's experience was a wake-up call for Peter and me. Soon after we laid my father to rest, we did something that we have always talked about doing but never got around to: we sat down and wrote out our wills. Both of us are embarrassed that it took us so long, because we're smart and not having wills is just plain stupid. But our lawyer isn't surprised by our inaction. While all parents should have one, he says, many simply put it off and eventually forget about it. Nine times out of ten, he tells us, it's fine and nothing sudden happens, so there's no harm. When I tell him what happened with my mom and the life insurance, he says that's not uncommon either. "She's not the first wife who let her husband handle all the money and she won't be the last." That may be true, but Peter and I aren't about to make the same mistake. Besides drawing up wills, our estate planning includes a review of life insurance policies, which reveals we could use a bit more.

Bottom line: money matters. And it matters whether you make a six-figure income or are barely scraping by. If you have children, it matters even more. Avoid making assumptions about how much (or how little) money you have. If you let a spouse or partner handle ongoing money chores like bill paying, banking, and insurance, don't check out: monitor it often. Don't bury your head on money issues. Be aware of every dollar that comes in and out. Every woman should have a handle on the finances that impact her and never assume that someone else has it covered and there's no need to be up on the specifics. It's not enough just to know each month how much comes in and where it's spent. Think more long-term, too: life insurance, disability coverage, health care, guardianships, wills, and estate planning. It's the unsexiest, most boring stuff, but absolutely essential. And it's easier to discuss the *what if*s when the emotional current is low than when you're in a crisis.

Never apologize for wanting to know every detail about your personal and household finances.

Celebrate Often

14

The sleeping man next to me never wears a stitch of clothing to bed. I think he's as handsome now as he was when I married him twenty years ago, despite some additional pounds on his frame. He's put up with a lot from me in recent months, this man who some friends describe as a cross between Russell Crowe and George Clooney.

Hmmm. It's early still, the kids have yet to stir in their rooms, and our bedroom door is shut. Marly is passed out on his little green L.L.Bean bed on the floor, perhaps dreaming of chasing rabbits. As I gently wake the sleeping man with a technique all my own, he doesn't resist.

"Happy anniversary," I say a few minutes later.

"Indeed!" Peter whispers.

I can't believe we've been married for twenty years. Some couples we know mark their wedding anniversaries alone, with quiet, romantic dinners at out-of-the-way restaurants. Not us. In our family, we party together and celebrate all milestones with one another. We've found that the more we celebrate, the more we have to celebrate.

For our Big 2-0, Emma researches restaurants, and true to her personality, checks out all the cool and hip places in Manhattan. She chooses one that she thinks we'll all like: Quality Italian on West 57th Street, midway between Tiffany & Co. and Carnegie Hall.

"Actually, Mom, I've wanted to go there since it opened, but it's expensive. Since everyone likes Italian and it's your big day, it's okay, right?"

"Of course, baby," I tell her.

That night we take a taxi to the restaurant, where we find Peter's son, Nick, waiting out front, looking as cool as ever. I met Nick when he was just seven. He came to live with us at age eleven and has been with us ever since. He is now twenty-eight and a graphic designer in Brooklyn, where he lives in a studio apartment above a busy butcher shop. He is a joy to be with—funny, smart, and considerate—and Emma and Jake idolize their older brother. In some ways, Nick has replaced my dad as their inveterate teaser, with emails and texts flying between Brooklyn and Manhattan at all hours. The kids love nothing better than to engage in a prolonged sassy exchange with Nick the Boss.

He hands me an envelope. It's clearly not an anniversary card. No, this is a business envelope and inside is a check for $2,000, a sum Nick asked to borrow several months before. I make a move to give it back, but he refuses to take it. "I asked for a loan, not a gift," he says. "I insist on repaying my debt."

This blows me away. Nick has always been an exceptional big brother to Jake and Emma, and they hang on his every word. But what never fails to move me is how true to his word he is, like now. I know he could use the money and that repaying me is no doubt a big stretch for him. But he does it anyway. Peter and I sometimes jokingly call him "GB." That's short for "good boy," which he knows is a term of endearment because it's what Peter always calls Marly. But Nick *is* a good boy, and we couldn't be more proud of him.

Every time we go out to dinner, especially at a place where food is bound to be plentiful, I steel myself to be strong, to stick to my low-carb regimen. My eating history is such that when I fall off the wagon, I tumble hard and it rarely lasts just one night. So I refuse to test myself and go there. But tonight I'm not cheating, I'm indulging with really good food and perfect company as I celebrate two decades of marriage to the man I love.

Emma and I share a plate of chicken parmesan that comes pizza shaped, big and round with melted mozzarella cheese and tomato sauce oozing all over the inch-thick chicken cutlet that is buried underneath. It's served with a bowl of arugula and various other toppings like drizzled honey and hot pepper flakes, but we add nothing because it tastes great the way it is. The three boys devour charred steaks. We eat so much food that nobody thinks of dessert. We're stuffed and every bite is absolutely worth it.

This dinner is a great reminder that no matter who we are or what we do, no matter how significant our accomplishments, what counts is the quality of our relationships with the people closest to us. Late that night, I tell Peter that our dinner made me so proud of our family. I feel really good about myself and us as a couple.

"These have been my best twenty years," Peter says. "And I bet the next twenty will be just as good or even better."

A few months later in the fall, a surprise party that I've planned to celebrate Peter's sixtieth birthday almost gets derailed by his grief over the sudden death of a friend.

"It was the saddest and most depressing morning ever," Peter says after returning from Connecticut on that cold, rainy October day. "It broke my heart."

"Should I cancel tonight?" I say, referring to the work event I had told him we've been invited to by a potentially big client.

"No," Peter says. "This is important for you. You're on a roll."

Peter met Paul White when they were undergrads at Syracuse, and they became fast friends. Over the past forty years, he's watched Paul's once promising life gradually but steadily decline. It ends in tragedy when he kills himself.

Paul was a rich prep school kid from Greenwich, Connecticut. After college, he quickly wowed Madison Avenue as a hotshot ad man at magazines like *Rolling Stone* and *Vanity Fair*. A dashing prince of the city, Paul dressed in finely tailored Paul Stuart suits with his signature silk pocket squares. But in the 1980s, one fling too many resulted in an unwanted pregnancy and the subsequent birth of a daughter. Within a few years, his life began to unravel. By the early '90s, Paul was drummed out of ad sales. He struggled with alcohol and drugs and had a contentious relationship with his young daughter's mom. To make ends meet, he began to sell art and antiques at the iconic Twenty-Sixth Street Flea Market and came to specialize in gently used upscale designer clothing and handbags. Paul was the only dealer who wore a blazer to the market each week, and certainly the only one with a pocket square. He did well catering to well-heeled clients looking for a deal.

Early in our marriage, Peter's child support payments cut deeply into his salary and we hit upon a way to make extra money. My mom had plenty of antiques left over from her closed business, and her friend Sandy orchestrated estate sales in Miami Beach. Voilà: a steady source of collectibles and antiques. We took a booth near Paul at Twenty-Sixth Street, and Peter supplemented his *USA Today* salary by selling at that market and at various antiques shows. He worked most weekends throughout the '90s and into the new millennium and did well enough to warrant a few buying trips to England. Network executives, producers, and anchors he covered would hear about Peter's side gig and often begin interviews with him by asking, "How's the antiques business?" He and Paul sold near each other for years. But by 2003, Women For Hire was doing well enough that I told Peter he didn't have to sell any more if he didn't want to.

"You don't have to twist my arm," Peter said as he abruptly—and gladly—traded weekends at the market for time with our family.

But Peter continues to head off to Twenty-Sixth Street pretty much every Saturday morning with Jake in tow, this time as a buyer, not a seller, and he invariably winds up spending the last half hour or so talking to his old friend Paul. When Peter tries to broach the subject of Paul's sobriety, which they'd talked about before, Paul waves him off and assures him he's okay. Then Paul stops coming to the flea market and a few days later

Peter learns he is dead. He was only sixty-three and Peter weeps when he hears the news. I can count on one hand the times I've seen him cry like that—and it breaks my heart.

Paul's death proved to be the second time in a year that Peter lost a close friend. Only nine months earlier his friend Jacques le Sourd had died. They met in the late 1970s at their first newspaper jobs, one a very gay man, the other very straight. Fast-forward to 2009 and Jacques gets laid off without warning after thirty-five years as Gannett Westchester's theater critic. His dismissal sends him adrift. Disbelief and deep depression replace his identity and his paycheck, and he blows through his meager life savings. Evicted from his apartment, he flees to England, where an old friend takes him in. The coroner says it was a heart attack, but those who loved Jacques know better: a pink slip cut him down at age sixty-four.

His *New York Times* obituary recalls a conversation with a colleague after he got his walking papers. "I was working on a story about the theater industry's financial woes: the Depression hits Broadway," Jacques said. "I don't have to do that story now. I'm living it."

Peter has grieved for Jacques all year and is reminded of him constantly. The sight of Hermès ties, which both Jacques and Paul favored; a mention of a hit Broadway show; or reading a Sunday "Styles" piece in the *New York Times* about older people finding or losing love later in life. "I've got no money, no prospects, no nothing," Jacques said in their last conversation. Peter overnighted some cash and was reaching out to friends in England to see if they could help when word of his death came. Had it not been for me and my businesses and our marriage, Peter said glumly, he might have faced Jacques's fate, too, after he took the buyout.

But now in the taxi Peter is thinking solely of Paul. "The saddest thing is knowing that one of your closest friends was in such pain, that he felt that his life was so worthless that ending it was his best option. It doesn't get much worse than that."

"You want to skip this thing?" I ask again.

"No, of course not. I can put on my happy face," Peter says.

Imagine his surprise then—an absolutely wonderful surprise—when he is greeted by sixty-five of his closest friends and family at The Press Lounge, an aptly named rooftop hot spot in a trendy boutique hotel overlooking the Hudson River. A minute earlier, I had texted Emma to say we'd arrived and to have everyone shout "Happy Birthday" when Peter walked through the door. For months, Peter has said he didn't want anything special for his birthday and would rather put the money in the college fund. But milestones are important, and we can't ignore his sixtieth. If we've learned anything this year, it's that we need to celebrate the good times while we can or live to regret it. Splurging on this party is well worth it and to see the genuine look of joy and gratitude on Peter's face is priceless.

Nick, Emma, and Jake give short toasts. Emma says that her dad has made his children promise to describe him at his funeral "as the funniest guy we have ever met. Well, while you're still above ground, Daddy, let's just set the record straight: you are in fact the funniest man we have ever met." Jake talks about Peter's affinity for cleanliness and his so-called ZT (zero-tolerance) policy of making sure the house is tidied up before they leave for school. And his thriftiness: "He comes into our rooms while we're semi-awake and picks up every piece of clothing that has pockets and shakes it down for quarters. When we ask why he's in desperate need for laundry money at this hour he says, 'Oh no, this is for your college fund.'"

Nick is next. "In the Johnson family, you learn to memorize *The Godfather*. There are three things that my dad has constantly reminded me of: Never tell anybody outside the family what you're thinking. Don't ever take sides with anyone against the family. And most importantly: a man who doesn't spend time with his family can never be a real man. It's all about family and my dad is a living testament to that. Happy birthday, Dad. We love you. Here's to the next sixty."

Peter is clearly moved and pauses before speaking. His voice quivering, he says: "It's a really dark day when you bury a friend who dies too early. That's what I did today. Life can be hard, and it's easy to think about the adversity we all face and how dark things can be. But we also have to cherish life and celebrate it. Times like this make life so worth living. I love all of you and am lucky to have the greatest family and friends." The crowd gives him a warm round of applause and Peter adds, "By the way, this is the last time any of you will see me tear up." Everyone laughs.

Watching Peter speak makes me wonder why I was ever anxious about him growing older. Thinking of Paul and Jacques, it reminds me of the saying "Don't regret getting older. It's a privilege denied to many." On the way home and for weeks afterwards, Peter's mood brightens considerably. "I never expected a party," he says. "I was absolutely blown away when I walked out on the deck and saw my dad standing there. To have all those people show up at a party for me is something I will never ever forget."

One day we're happy, healthy kids with smiles on our faces and the optimism of youth, with everything to look forward to. Then before we know it decades have passed and we're puffy faced, middle-aged, and either happy or sour. The choice is ours to make. We can believe that our dreams are long gone or unfulfilled and that our best years lie far, far behind us…or we can choose to believe the best is yet to come. I prefer to focus on one of my favorite sayings: "It's a good day to have a good day." The sudden death of Peter's dear friends, following on the heels of my father's equally sudden death, remind me of a line in *The Last Lecture*, by the late Carnegie Mellon professor Randy Pausch, who, like my dad, was diagnosed with pancreatic cancer. Unlike my dad, he knew his days were numbered and chose to live them fully, delivering extraordinary wisdom in a final university lecture that was turned into a book. He wrote, "The key question to keep asking is: Are you spending your time on the right things? Because time is all you have." I interpret that to include spending time with the right people, the ones who matter most to you, and never taking a moment for granted since all of this can be snatched away from each of us in a flash.

What counts in life is the quality of our relationships with the people closest to us.

15

Love the Ones You're With

've just finished my "Deals & Steals" segment with Michael Strahan, the newest addition to *Good Morning America*'s team. There seems to be nothing he can't handle, and he's even more gracious off-air than on. No wonder everyone from truck drivers and sports fans to stay-at-home moms and movie stars loves him. He is the real deal.

We bonded immediately during our first segment together a few months ago: Twenty seconds before our "Deals" segment begins, I realize he's been given a handheld microphone. That would be fine except that he needs both hands to lift and toss the gold boxes that cover each of my products to reveal what's underneath. Even an ex–New York Giant, Hall-of-Fame defensive end needs two free hands to juggle boxes and handle props without looking awkward and knocking around that mic. I signal one of the stagehands to grab the handheld and alert the audio team to use Michael's clip-on mic instead. All of that happens in an instant. A mini crisis has been averted, all of which Michael takes in silently. But when we finish the segment, he gives me an appreciative bear hug. He always exudes endless warmth and energy by reacting enthusiastically to each item I feature. Three minutes of joy.

As I walk into my office later, I think about how fortunate I am to work with such good people. The team at *GMA* includes the most dedicated, hardest-working people I have ever known. I'm just as blessed to have close friends who are always there for me, who have no ties to the glitz and glamour of the network news industry. It's comforting to know that I benefit in so many ways from women I see infrequently but text often. We all know we're there for each other 24/7 and would drop everything in a flash if one of us needed help.

Some years ago my friend Cindy's father had emergency bypass surgery in Lubbock, Texas, and she rushed from her home in Tulsa to be at his side. Cindy and I had worked closely together at my Spark & Hustle conferences, and I could tell from her voice on the phone that she was very worried her dad might not make it.

On a whim I got on a plane and flew to Dallas and then took a short flight to Lubbock. On my way to surprise her at the hospital I asked the cabdriver—the one I waited forty-five minutes for since there's no line of waiting taxis at the Lubbock airport like there is in New York—where I could buy fresh flowers. "That would be Walmart, ma'am," he said. It felt good seeing the look of shock and appreciation on Cindy's face when I walked into that small community hospital to cheer her up, flowers in hand. Whenever she talks about me, Cindy invariably mentions the time I traveled all the way to Texas to be with her family for a few hours before making the trip home the same day. But the truth is that I know she'd do the same for me.

The night after the mic incident at *GMA*, Peter and I have dinner with our old friends Nina and Jim. Jim and I go way back. We became friends when we both worked at NBC News—I was in PR, he was a producer. I introduced him to Peter, he introduced me to his wife, Nina, and the four of us have been friends ever since. Nina and I were pregnant at the same time, and their daughter, Natalie, is only a few months younger than Jake and Emma. When Natalie was an infant, they moved from New York to Montclair, New Jersey. It's just a little more than an eighteen-mile drive from Manhattan to Montclair, but after they moved, we all busied ourselves in family and work and lost touch for a number of years. But now that the kids are getting ready to head off to college, we decide it's time to get back together.

"You look great," Jim says to me with a big hug and a kiss, which Nina repeats a few seconds later.

Nina gets right to the point. "What's the best part of losing so much weight?"

Before I can answer, Peter jumps in: "The best part is that she's finally stopped saying—" but Nina interrupts, "'Not tonight, honey, because I don't *feel good* about my body'?" Everyone laughs. We spend the next couple of hours in the upper level of a popular theater district bistro, away from the busy bar. It's perfect because the four of us think alike about all sorts of issues and can speak freely without having to worry about offending anyone at the table. It takes just moments for us to pick up where we left off years ago: finishing each other's sentences, sharing parenthood tales, and catching up on work, life, and media industry gossip.

It's rare when two couples get together and all four people like each other equally. Often, as Peter and I have discovered, someone in the foursome ends up being the odd one out. Or perhaps the women like each other but the men have nothing in common—or the other way around. Fortunately that's not the case with Nina and Jim. When it's finally time to say goodbye, we agree we all need to spend more time with each other and with the people we love.

During the cab ride home, Peter and I talk about how much fun we had and how much we regret not seeing them all those years; we were too busy being too busy—an easy crutch that I now regret. Reconnecting with old friends and nurturing new friendships is another thing that I pledge to put on my agenda. Peter is the outgoing, gregarious one, always ready to invite people over for dinner or to go out, but I'm more private. That must change because once the kids are away at school, staying busy, engaged, and connected with other people will take on more importance. Why face an empty nest alone with your spouse when there are all kinds of friendships out there, waiting to be rekindled?

Besides, the greatest joy in life is having dear friends and family to share it with. Everyone in our family agrees that one of the keys to happiness is staying mentally and physically active and engaging with many people. Now ninety-two, Peter's father, Jim, still takes the train in from Westchester to New York to see off-Broadway plays with Peter or any of his three daughters. Jim's dance card is full most days between movies, book clubs, Bible class, and lunches and dinners with a steady stream of old friends. If he worries about anything other than the obvious, he never lets on.

Surround yourself with people who make you feel good about yourself and who are there for you, even if you have limited interaction. We all have different friends for different reasons, of course, but there also comes a time when you need to tend to your friendship garden, weeding and pruning the stuff that has stopped growing and focus on that which continues to flower and bring you joy.

Vow to make kind people your kinda people.

A NEWER ME

Create the highest, grandest vision possible for
your life, because you become what you believe.
—*Oprah Winfrey*

Sit Less and Move More

16

For several months, I've been hinting rather broadly about wanting a treadmill desk without taking the plunge and actually buying one. After all, it would be a perfect complement to my ongoing healthy-living-weight-loss plan, which has been super simple from the start. I have just three areas of focus: eat less, choose better, move more. The first two were initially challenging. But the third, moving more, was a snap since I barely moved *at all*. A walk around the block felt like a major victory in the early days. Eventually I joined a gym, took up jogging with the kids in Central Park a couple times a week, and, most days, spent twenty to thirty minutes on the treadmill in my bedroom.

But while all that sounds good on paper—and I monitor my daily activity with a wristband tracker—I still have what experts politely call a "sedentary lifestyle." Unless I'm traveling and on the go, I sit for eight to ten hours a day, like millions of people do every single day.

I begin to read more about the hazards of sitting. Dr. James Levine of the Mayo Clinic coins the adage "Sitting is the new smoking." He says that by planting ourselves in front of computers all day we increase our risk of diabetes, heart disease, and cancer. Worse, research indicates that a dose of exercise here and there doesn't undo the damage created by a whole day of sitting.

Yikes.

Then a study in the *Journal of the National Cancer Institute* brings the message home: For every two hours of sitting, our risk of lung cancer rises six percent, colon cancer eight percent, and endometrial cancer ten percent. I didn't seek out this information, but as I read it I start suggesting to Peter that a treadmill desk might be in my future.

One morning a month or so later, after Peter and Marly and I walk the fourteen blocks from home to the office, I find that my desk has been removed. In its place is a new sleek treadmill desk.

"Cheers to the last twenty years and to our next twenty," Peter says of this belated anniversary present. Having struggled for two decades to find appropriate birthday, Valentine's, anniversary, and Christmas gifts for his oh-so-picky wife, he has hit a home run. It's exactly what I'd been hoping for.

This treadmill desk has a glass top forty-five inches above the floor supported by two metal pedestals. The treadmill itself is separate and slides easily under the desk. There are no drawers, which forces me to go through my old desk drawers and throw away stuff I've accumulated but haven't touched in years.

Peter carts off my comfy, perfectly worn-in high-back leather IKEA chair. I have a momentary flash of panic when it occurs to me that the novelty of this nifty new machine could fade quickly, like every other piece of exercise equipment I've ever owned. I worry I'll wind up donating it to a more worthy recipient, or just putting it out on the street, which is what happened years ago when I got the exercise bug and impulsively bought a NordicTrack, then an elliptical. Both became expensive coatracks then giveaways to our building employees before I settled on a treadmill in our bedroom that our whole family actually uses for its intended purpose.

But my new treadmill desk is different. The first few days of standing and walking and typing on a keyboard—all at the same time—takes some getting used to. But unlike an elliptical or NordicTrack, it's pretty hard to ignore a treadmill desk because it requires so little effort to use. It's now my only desk, so I have no choice but to use it. Unlike a traditional treadmill, this machine has a maximum speed of only three miles an hour. For me, setting it at just under two miles an hour works best, which is the norm according to the instruction manual. It's a fairly slow, steady walking pace, and on an average day in the office, I log at least five miles. I don't walk all day; I like to mix it up, alternating walking with standing still so I don't get tired or bored. Five miles a day is twenty-five miles a week or well over one thousand miles a year, miles that I would never accomplish without the help of this machine. I can't help but believe there's got to be some health benefit from it.

Standing up most of the day becomes my new normal. For starters, I can't sit down because my chair is gone, but once I get used to standing all day the thought of sitting becomes somewhat foreign. I post photos on Facebook of myself at my treadmill desk and I write about it in a full-page feature in the

New York Post. Good Morning America does a little segment about it where Robin and I are walking on treadmills in the middle of Times Square. A few days later I am walking at the same treadmill desk with the ladies on *The View*. The reaction is mixed: lots of interest, but most people are convinced that they could never get used to it. They assume it takes advanced coordination to walk and work. Trust me, it doesn't. When I travel around the country speaking about my Shift, one of the things I tell every woman I meet is *If I can lose weight, anyone can*. This is the same deal. If I, a recovering couch potato, can walk and talk and type at the same time and actually enjoy it, anyone can. It's not hard.

In her book *The First 20 Minutes*, Gretchen Reynolds, who is the phys ed columnist for the *New York Times*, writes that research shows that even regular exercisers may not be doing enough to counteract the health hazards of sitting at a desk all day long.

"Sitting for long periods of time—when you don't stand up, don't move at all—tends to cause changes physiologically within your muscles," she told *Fresh Air*'s Terry Gross on National Public Radio. "You stop breaking up fat in your bloodstream, you start getting accumulations of fat…in your liver, your heart, and your brain. You get sleepy. You gain weight. You basically are much less healthy than if you're moving."

She recommends standing for two minutes every twenty minutes while deskbound, even if you can't move around your office. "That sounds so simple, but it actually has profound consequences. If you can stand up every twenty minutes, even if you do nothing else, you change how your body responds physiologically."

Clearly, not all workspaces are conducive to treadmill desks. But with health-care costs skyrocketing and companies becoming more focused on keeping their workforce healthier, treadmill desks will become commonplace in more corporate environments. If your company says no to a treadmill desk, there are other ways to get off your butt: when you're on the phone, make sure you're on your feet. Take the stairs whenever you can; there are seventy steps to our fourth-floor office and I try to use them whenever I'm coming or going. If I climb the stairs twice a day, five days a week, that's seven hundred steps a week for doing nothing but skipping the elevator—and every one of them counts toward my ten-thousand-a-day goal. Speaking of steps, get yourself a tracker or use an app to measure your movement. The latest iPhones have built-in step trackers.

All of this—the desks, the trackers, the emphasis on walking more and sitting less—comes at a time when we are more sedentary than ever. It's so easy to plop ourselves down in front of the computer and never get up. If you work at home, you might consider looking into a treadmill desk. I'm buoyed whenever I hear from people who inquire about my model (**RebelDesk.com**), but there is a wide variety of manufacturers to choose from.

If this former couch potato can walk and work at the same time, you can, too.

17

Change Your Hair

Y ou look like Nancy Grace."

I thought that once I lost weight I'd stop getting feedback from viewers who say I should be ashamed for letting myself go and embarrassed to look like a blob on national TV. Instead, armchair stylists at home continue to advise me to stop wearing black or complain that my voice annoys them or that my hair looks terrible. The enabling power of the Web and the courage it gives people to email and say whatever they want, often bluntly and cruelly, continues to astound me. When we read comments from Internet trolls, Emma is the first to say, "Haters gonna hate," which is code for "Consider the source and brush it off."

But Dora Smagler, one of ABC's top hair stylists, is no hater and she greets me with that Nancy Grace jab the second I walk into *Good Morning America*'s hair and makeup room about an hour before my live segment. At that moment we see Nancy on the TV monitor next to the mirror in front of us, talking to ABC News legal analyst Dan Abrams about the crime du jour. Dora and I burst out laughing because she's right: both

Nancy and I share the same color and the exact same "helmet" shape hairdo, but it works for just one of us. Only Nancy can do Nancy.

On my journey from feeling fed up to fabulous, I've changed things about my lifestyle and attitude that no longer worked in my favor. I hadn't thought about changing my hair but apparently my bosses have, which prompts Dora's comment.

For the second time during my years on the program, the bigwigs have ideas on improving my appearance. I'm a little apprehensive, but nowhere near the panic I felt when I discovered they wanted me to lose weight. I get it: TV is a visual medium and producers want viewers to like what they see, which is why they sweat the details like the hair style of a weekly contributor. It's business, not personal. But I'm slightly taken aback because I hadn't anticipated this conversation, and I have a live segment coming up. I tell Dora there's no time to transform me in the moments I have.

"Oh yes, there is," she says, guiding me into the chair, putting a cape around my neck, and snapping it into place. Ordinarily I wouldn't let anyone touch my hair on the spot, but I trust Dora, so I let her do her thing. She gets to work instantly and her hands move quickly and effortlessly. She divides my hair into sections with a few clips, snips some here and there, and generally messes it up. It takes all of six minutes, which she knows is all the time we have since I must get down to the studio.

"You don't want it to look so perfectly coifed," she tells me. "Lose the lacquer hair spray and allow it to move naturally."

With that, she places a mirror in my hand and spins the chair around so I get a full view of the front and back. "I love it. It's me, only looser," I say.

"Figured you would," Dora says, giving me a hug as she assures me she'll help me get it just right. "This is just a rapid re-do." Dora is brutally honest when it comes to hair. She doesn't sugarcoat what she thinks looks good and what doesn't, which is why many ABC News correspondents trust her and only her to cut and style their hair.

Dora also tells me that the show runners think I'll look better as a brunette with subtle blond highlights. "Don't worry," she says, "the color will happen later today," but I beg off, saying that my afternoon is packed with meetings and there's no way I can do it. Yet the truth is that no matter how much I respect Dora, I'm wary of a color change, having been blonde forever. I need some time to process the idea. Growing up, I always admired iconic blondes, from Marilyn Monroe to Diane Sawyer. The most obvious word attached to "blonde" is "bombshell." That's most definitely not me, but I am a natural blonde and I have childhood photos to prove it. As a teenager driving around Miami Beach in my aging black convertible with its fading, cracked gray leather interior, my hair naturally lightened from the direct sun, helped by generous spritzes of Sun-In. I loved the image of being blonde in a beach community, the whole fun-in-the-sun thing, and it never occurred to me that I could or should be anything else. When my hair began to darken in college, I started to get highlights. In my thirties, my hairdresser made it even lighter.

Looking at photos of us at a friend's wedding years ago, I can't help but cringe at how washed-out my hair looks. It has virtually no contrast, which as I look at it now, is neither stylish nor flattering. Neither is the black tent I am wearing, which at the time I felt hid my weight but which I now realize only accentuated it and certainly fooled no one.

"How do you feel about it?" Peter asks later at home when I tell him I'm to be a brunette.

I pause for a second, weighing what I want to say to him. I have to admit that changing my hair color intrigues me. Maybe it's because I'm going through this period of personal transition and thinking hard about so many things. Or maybe I'm too focused on that stuff to get too worked up about my hair.

"I think some changes can be good," I finally say.

"Sounds like you're on the fence," he says.

"Cut to the chase," I say. "What do you think about having a brunette as a wife?"

"Might be nice to have the curtains match the carpet," he says, mugging, as I slug his arm.

The bosses seem to want my color fixed ASAP, so the next day I meet Dora at the famed Louis Licari Salon in midtown, fifteen floors above bustling Fifth Avenue. Erika, a colorist with a deep roster of TV clients, takes it slowly. She's petite with a soft voice, but no pushover: this girl kicks butt several times a week at Spin class and when it comes to color, she pulls no punches either. She tells me that she knows that going from blonde to brunette is a massive change, but not to worry. "I'm in your hands," I say.

Nearly twenty years of highlighting with blond streaks every six weeks has cost me dearly with thinning, over-processed hair, not to mention what it has done to my bank account. Dora assures me that those days are over and that the darker color will more closely resemble my natural color. She says my hair will be healthier and shine on TV. Double benefits, maybe even triple. I trust her.

Erika mixes the formula and applies it to my hair. But after she rinses and towel-dries, both she and Dora reject it. "Still too light. Keep going…darker, much darker," Dora says as Erika nods in agreement. Erika looks at me to gauge my reaction. I tell her to go for it, figuring they know best. Erika continues to adjust the base, carefully painting the front strands with a lighter blond, which come out too stripy. She fiddles for nearly four hours until they're both satisfied.

When we had arrived at the salon, Dora showed me a photo of a random girl's dark brown ponytail and said that was her vision for me. It seemed far-fetched at the time, but now that color is my new reality. Dora asks if I resent her for doing this.

"No, no way, not at all," I say. "I'm grateful that you care."

Still unsure, she prods, "Promise?"

"Absolutely," I assure her.

It not only looks more natural, it somehow feels more natural, too. I don't overthink it. The next week at *Good Morning America*, Robin notices immediately. "I love what you've done," she says, beaming, during a break. "It looks sensational and suits you well."

I'm sold and relieved to reaffirm that change *is* good. French fashion icon Coco Chanel once said, "A woman who cuts her hair is about to change her life." I never thought I'd look good with darker hair, which is why I stayed so light all these years. But with the change I start to get compliments from all around. The best line comes from Jake. As a preoccupied-with-all-kinds-of-things teenage boy, he would be the last one in our house to notice any deviation in his mom's hair. "You look so much younger, mom," he says matter-of-factly a couple weeks after my redo. "You and Emma could be sisters." A bit of an exaggeration, no doubt, but his words make me feel good and along with my new look, put an unexpected psychological spring in my step.

Change can be daunting, but it can also make you feel great. Shaking it up and doing something new to your hair is one of the easiest ways to give yourself a fresh start—a simple mental reset. Whether you do your own hair color at home or head to a salon and allow a stylist to take charge, give yourself the freedom to imagine new possibilities. I discovered that one of the best things about changing hair style or the color is that it's not permanent: time will fix a mistake. And if you want a big change on a minimal budget, call your local hairstyling school: they often look for clients who students can refine their skills on under the watchful eyes of instructors.

Change can be good. Don't let the fear of it stop you from experimenting.

See Yourself Through a Stylist's Eyes

18

On *Ellen*, comedian Amy Schumer says Los Angeles is the only city where her arms register as legs. It gets a laugh, and that's me in a nutshell. My upper arms are as big as some women's thighs, or so I think, which is why in moments of weakness I sometimes secretly refer to myself as a four-legged woman. I hate my flabby biceps, so much so that I never wear sleeveless dresses. Never ever, as Taylor Swift would say. I suppose I could go to a gym and lift weights to tone those biceps, but I'm fairly sure that'll never happen. What can I say?

Many women in America have the same problem, yet for some reason the vast majority of designers primarily manufacture sleeveless dresses. I've never understood why, and when I complain about it to Adam Glassman, the creative director of *O, the Oprah magazine*, he understands immediately. There was a time in my life when counting a member of Oprah's dream team as a trusted friend would have been a stretch. But that's what we've become after I first invited Adam to appear with me on *Good Morning America* for several special "Deals & Steals" segments featuring his boss's favorite things. He knows better than to suggest a sweater or shrug, as the extra layer adds unwanted bulk. Instead, he tells me to contact my favorite designer to ask if I can buy extra fabric to have sleeves made.

As Oprah's not-so-secret design weapon, Adam knows every trick. I reach out to the public relations team at Lafayette 148, and much to my surprise they say yes, they can assist. Obviously they're not dummies: it can't hurt to help a regular *Good Morning America* contributor look better on the air. But with clients from Oprah to Michelle Obama, they don't need my business, which makes their response even more impressive to me. After Lafayette adds sleeves to one of their sleeveless dresses and I wear it on TV and tag it on Instagram, the company says they get a number of calls from women asking how they can order the same dress. If enough of us speak up, my dilemma may be resolved in a season or two, or so I hope.

The lesson is: If you don't ask, you'll never know.

I got more comfortable with my wardrobe choices after an unexpected session with a professional stylist. During The Chat—the one that precipitated *The Shift*—Barbara Fedida had said she wanted to send me to a stylist, a suggestion I reacted to in horror because I was convinced that her words were code for *you are fat*. I never took her up on her offer because I knew at the time that no matter what I wore, it wouldn't hide the fact that I needed to lose weight.

But after my Shift, she offers again.

"No pressure at all and it's my gift to you," she says. "We have an amazing new stylist now who everybody loves and I just want you to have the experience." There was a time not so long ago when such a remark would send a shiver down my spine; I'd be convinced that she still thought I dressed like a frump.

But at this point, I am dramatically lighter than I was when Barbara and I first met, having dropped several sizes. The suggestion doesn't feel so fraught this time around, so I'm game. The stylist is Karyn Starr, a doe-eyed beauty with flawless skin, chestnut-brown hair, and a fit body beneath her loose-fitting, premium designer clothes. The first time we meet, she comes to my apartment to look in my closet. She starts by asking me to show her what I love most. Then she dives right in with her critique. She doesn't fool around.

"You can give this away," she says as she points to a cutesy heart-patterned silk shirt. "And this, too," she says of a top that she clearly thinks is unflattering for my body type. Looking at a soft leather jacket, she tells me, "This is great with jeans and a tank for date night." And finally: "I like this for casual Sundays. Try this on and let's see the fit." She comments pleasantly but firmly about everything in my closet, stopping first to ask how I think I look my best, wanting to genuinely understand how I see myself. We put the clothes she says aren't flattering on me in a pile; it will head to Housing Works, a thrift shop down the street that benefits people living with HIV and AIDS.

Then the real fun begins: We are off to department stores. Karyn makes it clear up front that there's no pressure on me to buy a thing. She is not on commission and ABC is paying for her time, so there's no hard sell, just *Let's try this on!* She steers me away from loose, oversize clothes by showing me that I can wear not only fitted pieces but also different fabrics and cuts, stripes and patterns that I long thought were off-limits. "If a piece goes up to your neck," she says, "be sure to expose your wrists." She's big on pushing up sleeves, suggesting we alter one beautiful blazer with what she calls bracelet-length cuffs. In just a few hours, I learn that clothing options can be a joy, not a chore. She forces me to be more versatile with my choices. Her advice changes the way I think about clothes and, more specifically, how I view myself in them. I'm excited to make several purchases. After buying at two stores, I nix going to a third. "My budget's spent, Karyn," I declare. "Game over!"

I went into the process with the assumption that having a stylist is a wealthy person's luxury. I come away with a completely different perspective. There's a reason why nonprofit organizations like Dress for Success and Bottomless Closet— both of which focus on job readiness and economic independence for women—offer clients personalized sessions with stylists to assist with fresh wardrobe choices. They understand that the right clothing and accessories can boost a woman's confidence and sense of self-worth and make a significant difference in how she presents herself.

As Karyn shows me, it has little to do with designer labels or the price of a garment and everything to do with understanding the connection between fabrics, cuts, and varying body types. When a pro is there to help, not judge, a woman can see herself differently and gain a strong, fresh vision of her very best self. That is an eye-opener for me, especially since I always thought that I knew with certainty what worked and what didn't. I was wrong. The way you see yourself can be limiting, and the way others see you can open your mind to something completely different.

Nearly a year after my time with Karyn, I am about to leave the *Good Morning America* studio. I'm wearing a fitted dress with three-quarter-length sleeves that Karyn said looked good on me that day in my bedroom. I'm even comfortable wearing it without Spanx, which she prefers because comfort, not constriction, she says, is what fashion is all about. I'm also carrying a bright red bag. Between commercial breaks, anchor Lara Spencer stands at a mirror with her hairdresser, who is giving her a little fluff-up. Lara spots the bag, touches it, and then eyes the dress too as she runs her hand along my sleeve. She nods with approval and whispers to me, "You treat yourself right, girl."

As I head outside, I realize I *am* treating myself better, not just with a new bag every six months, or a new outfit, but in everything I do. I am deliberately focused on embracing all of me—inside and out.

Every woman should have a Karyn Starr experience at least once every few years. If you're reexamining yourself and working to improve your self-image, seek out a nonprofit with complimentary services or treat yourself to a stylist's time and expertise. In some cities, rates start as low as $25 an hour for a seasoned pro. When possible, avoid someone who is on commission, since she may be tempted to push pricy stuff or specific labels at you. And remember, you shouldn't have to buy a thing; just getting a new perspective can teach you so much. If you find the prospect of spending time with a stylist somewhat intimidating, ask a friend whose sense of style you admire to help you select outfits the next time you go shopping. My time with Karyn opened my mind to new options and ideas, which remain with me today. It is freeing and reassuring to discover that I can look and feel great in pieces that I would have walked right by and never tried on. It broadens my sense of what's possible.

> **Choose clothing and accessories that boost your confidence and self-worth.**

19

Wear Red Underwear

A publicist calls to thank me for featuring her client on "Deals & Steals." She says they've already gotten more than five thousand orders and it's only noon—they expect to sell far more by the time buying ends at midnight. We begin talking about other things and she says she's spending the afternoon prepping to pitch a new client the next day.

"Have any words of wisdom?" she asks.

"Wear red underwear," I say without hesitating.

"I'm down with that!" she says. But then she pauses and asks, "Why red underwear?"

I've always liked red underwear because I feel there's something that's simultaneously naughty and empowering about the color. I've advised more than a few women who need a psychological boost before heading into a high-stakes conversation to go red. It's a power color that you may not be able to pull off on the outside, but when you wear red underwear it's a hidden superpower that only *you* know about. When you're feeling down or unsure or nervous, put on some red undies and show the world who's boss. Wear red undies and you've got a good luck charm and a sure-fire confidence booster wrapped in one. My dresser drawer is filled with them.

As I build a stronger me, I realize I could use a new pair of red undies myself. I already have my neon yellow Nike sneakers, which Peter calls my "don't mess with me sneaks." When I wear them in the park, every step seems easier. To mark my accomplishment after my Shift, I had a small gold and diamond charm custom-made in the shape of the number 62 to signify my initial weight loss. It hangs from a bracelet on my left wrist and I never take it off, not even through airport security. It stays on me 24/7 and I rub it with my right hand whenever I'm in an intimidating or important situation. I view it as an integral part of my security arsenal that shields me from danger, the kind that can sometimes appear in the form of cupcakes. I'm always on the lookout for stuff like my bracelet to make me feel strong.

It doesn't take long before an opportunity to put my red underwear theory to the test presents itself. I am speaking at a conference in Long Beach, California. I've given hundreds of speeches in my life, but I've never stood alone on stage in front of thirteen thousand people, which is what I'm about to do for an entire hour. I am here to talk to direct sales reps for Nerium, a skin-care company, about personal and professional challenges and triumphs. The main event is in a cavernous arena where people fill the main floor and a balcony. Every seat is taken, yet somehow it feels intimate.

It's just me and thirteen thousand of my friends, hanging out. The last time I was here in the Long Beach Convention Center was in 2010 for Maria Shriver's California Women's Conference, which drew thousands of women. Her superstar husband, Arnold Schwarzenegger, was in his last term as governor and Oprah and Michelle Obama spoke from this same stage.

This time it's me alone. I can talk to five million *Good Morning America* viewers and not get nervous, but now I have twenty-six thousand eyes staring intently at me. The crowd is welcoming and gracious with laughter and applause as I speak about my own heartaches and successes. They're here for inspiration and they hang on every word.

I want to bottle the energy in this hall. It feels like this is my personal cheering squad—and it's thirteen thousand strong. Having my own peanut gallery, a core group of family and friends who root for me no matter what, has long been a source of strength. But for a while I withdrew from allowing them to support me, partially because I was embarrassed that I had temporarily lost my way. Never again. Being here is a reminder that I have a special squad that always has my back. These people can not only prevent me from failing, but they also push me to succeed.

When I start coughing midway through this speech and think I'm losing my voice, someone in the audience races from her seat to the stage to bring me bottled water and cough drops. As I take a sip and catch my breath, I hear women say from random parts of the balcony: "We love you, Tory. Take your time."

I love them right back, so much so that I take a risk: I ask everyone to stand so I can snap a selfie from the stage. I want to capture this magical memory. To up the ante, I ask them for their favorite mantras for a short video that I'll post on Facebook. They give me three and I choose one, guiding everyone in the convention center as they say in unison: "Two a day. I'm all in. See you on the cruise." It's their sales code that says when you commit to making two new connections a day, it shows you're all in and it may earn you a spot on an all-expenses-paid cruise.

Backstage, unbeknownst to me, Peter has recorded that moment on a monitor. He is blown away by the size of the crowd and what I've just done, so on a whim he sends the clip to several friends and relatives. He gets immediate feedback: *Tory is a rock star!*

As I walk offstage to a standing ovation, a barrage of texts appears on my phone from the people back home who have watched, courtesy of Peter's video. The best one comes from Barbara Fedida: "OMG. That looks like a Taylor Swift concert!" When I sign books for an hour and a half afterwards, the on-site bookseller tells me that every copy of *The Shift*, more than seven hundred books, has sold. I've got my mojo back again, just like when I first lost all that weight. This is a victory for me. It feels good to know that I'm back and that it shows. I'm not a rock star, but I feel like one today and I don't think it's a coincidence that I am wearing red underwear.

Put on a pair of red underwear and rock your confidence.

20

Declare Your Fabulousness

Just days after my red-undies conversation with the publicist, Emma shows some bravado when she makes a gutsy suggestion for a speech I'm about to give in Nashville. I've brought her along with me, and even though she's never been on stage, my seventeen-year-old is advising me on how to command the audience at the conference where I'll speak in a few hours. I let her talk because that's what moms do.

As I stand before the mirror in our Opryland hotel bathroom putting on makeup, Emma dares me to take the stage with my pinky and pointer fingers extended, with the others tucked down in the "rock on" stance.

She wants my opening words to be "I'm f***ing fabulous!"

"Why?" I ask. While the profanity is a turnoff, I'm genuinely puzzled as to *why* this phrase might appeal to my audience.

"You've got to show them who's boss, that you *own* the

crowd," Emma says, momentarily looking up from her iPhone, which never seems to leave her hand.

"How would using those particular words accomplish that?"

"Because nobody's going to mess with a woman who declares that she's f***ing fabulous," Emma says, explaining something so obvious to her clueless mom.

I adore Emma, but at this moment I think she's gone slightly mad. Or maybe it's just a kid fantasy to stand up and say such a thing, as if it's a wild concert. She might have a point, but a few hours later when I give the speech I don't include her suggested opener.

She teases me later on the way to dinner: "Ma, you're such a chicken."

"I wasn't afraid," I respond. "I just didn't understand what point it would have made."

"Sometimes I get the feeling that you don't think you're as great as you are, Mom," my blunt daughter says. "You have so much to be proud of and you should act like you know it."

I come away from her message—and the vibe I apparently gave off—determined to be more outwardly confident, just as I want her to be.

Like she does whenever we travel, Emma has already looked up Nashville's hot spots. She's skilled at picking winners. Her initial research leads to restaurants with a little too much southern for my comfort. Fried chicken sounds really good right about now—or anytime actually—but I'd rather not test my willpower, especially at the end of a long, exhausting day. By process of elimination, we land at Virago, supposedly the best sushi spot in town. We joke about how dramatically different our food choices are from our last Nashville visit, during Christmas break in 2011, which played a big role in the start of my Shift. No cheat meals this time, though. We don't touch the rice and say no when our waiter offers dessert. That is also a significant departure from our girls' week in Los Angeles a couple summers ago. The vacation where Emma and I went overboard at Millions of Milkshakes with a sugary concoction that contained more than a month's worth of carbs. In the moment it seemed like a good idea, worth every sip of chocolate goodness, until I panicked during the last slurp. It was downhill from there as I remember eating everything in sight. That trip became affectionately known as my Shift Storm and it taught me that staying away from empty carbs is a practice from which I should rarely deviate because for me that's key to continuing to lose weight.

Two weeks later Emma and I take off for Seattle. I am speaking at an Urban Campfire event designed to bring women together for candid conversation and TED-style talks. Emma's friend Lauren joins us from San Francisco at the W hotel downtown. She visited us in New York earlier in the year, and this is just the second time the girls have seen each other since they met on their month-long trip to Ecuador last summer.

The event is already underway inside a gigantic, twenty-thousand-square-foot former airplane hangar at Seattle's Magnuson Park. Emma reminds me that this is the last trip that she and I will take together before her high school senior year starts in September. "Look at this crowd, Mom! These are exactly the kind of women who would *love* to hear you take the stage and declare exactly who you are." Clearly, Emma is on a mission. She eggs me on, aided by her co-conspirator, Lauren, who is a year older and heading to college in the fall. The stage is round, with the audience on all sides, so speakers walk in circles to make eye contact with everyone there. During my introduction, Emma softly whispers, "Do it, Mom. Make me proud."

I take my spot on the stage, surrounded by hundreds of women, and get right to it.

"My daughter, Emma, has dared me to let you all in on a little secret. So here goes. No more shrinking violet, no more playing small when we are meant to rule the world."

I pause for a beat. It's too late to turn back now. Then forcefully and confidently I say, "I am f***ing fabulous!"

The applause is deafening, uplifting and powerful. I see through the corner of my eye that Emma and Lauren are jumping up and down, high-fiving each other. It's their victory: They got me to do it and are oh-so-proud of themselves. I'm happy for them both, but particularly Emma.

At the end of my speech, I take a few questions. One woman suggests that Emma come onstage and reenact what she dared *me* to do. In the wings, I spot Emma shaking her head and mouthing *No way!* But the audience will have none of it and starts chanting her name. There's no hiding now. Emma walks forward sheepishly. Not only is it the first time that she and I have ever shared a stage, but it's the first time she's even spoken before an audience larger than her classroom.

Emma grabs the mic and I count her down: "Three, two, one…"

"I'm f***ing fabulous!" she roars, as proudly as she can. The women give her a standing ovation and Lauren greets her in the wings with a bear hug for her bestie. That's my girl. "I told you they would love it, Mom," Emma says later over dinner, probably the fifth time since the event. "I thought it was a cool idea, but to tell you the truth, I was kind of worried it'd bomb," Lauren says. "What if they had responded with silence?"

"I knew that wouldn't happen because if you declare who you are, as long as you believe it, that's enough," Emma says. I marvel at their maturity. The girls quickly move on like the teens they are, obsessing between themselves about what to order for dinner. It gives me time to ponder what was just said. It's true: If the story we tell ourselves is one of inadequacy, of never being enough, of never having enough, then that becomes our reality. But if we believe that we are fabulous and that we are indeed enough in all ways, and that we have enough, then *that* is the life we live.

That night back at the hotel, Emma plugs her iPhone into a stereo speaker, turns up the volume on Katy Perry's "Roar," and the three of us break into dance. Going wild like this is something Emma and I got into a few years ago, knowing that movement can dramatically improve our mood at the end of a long day. Plus, it's exercise that doesn't feel like a chore. We're already on a high from this day, but you never need an excuse to dance, especially when no one is looking.

Lauren, getting ready to start her freshman semester at Portland State, says she's pretty sure that this trip taught her more about life and what's truly important than anything she learned in high school. "It *was* f***ing fabulous," she says.

When the girls are asleep in the bed next to me, I think of the gift they gave me today. They urged me to do something bold, to take a leap of faith in myself. Being content gives me the confidence to share and celebrate who I am. Theatrics and dares aside, I *am* f***ing fabulous and I'm glad I had the courage to say it out loud. It's very different from the slump I was in just months earlier, when declaring that I was awesome would have definitely been a massive stretch. Now I am ready to stand up for myself, to speak up for myself. It is something that all of us should be able to do anytime.

We're all on a journey to discover our inner fabulous, or as Emma would say, our inner *f***ng* fabulous. We fool ourselves into thinking it's about our weight, hair, and makeup. But it's really about our smiles, hearts, and guts. It's about the promises we make to ourselves, and the commitment it takes to keep them. It's about the compassion we show ourselves if and when we slip up along the way.

Stand up and declare to the world that you are fabulous.

21

Every Girl Needs
a Tiara

My mom and dad bought their home in Miami Beach in 1974, when I was four years old. The house is a white stucco ranch, built in the early '50s. The structure itself doesn't look like much, so my mom took the lead on interior style and décor by painting the walls in eye-popping reds and yellows, laying down leopard-print carpet accented by classic black leather and chrome chairs, Art Deco lamps, and vintage wood and silver accessories throughout. When I was in college, they added a lap pool in the backyard and planted large palm trees and other tropical foliage. My father loved to work in the yard, transplanting trees and bushes, growing orchids, and creating a stylized jungle look. Sitting in the Jacuzzi next to the pool, you felt that Tarzan could swing by at any moment.

My fondest memories of the house are all the family gatherings with grandparents, aunts, uncles, cousins, and close friends. Virtually every holiday is an excuse for my mom to

throw a party. Daytime ones are informal, with kids wet from
the pool running in and out of the house. Nighttime affairs are
more formal, a perfect excuse to dress up the dining room with
embroidered linen tablecloths (never paper), vintage china,
and sterling silverware (never plastic) and crystal glasses (not
red Solo cups). Day or night, my mom serves stone crabs from
Joe's, filet mignon, and fist-size shrimp. She stages desserts on
antique glass cake plateaus and muffin baskets and hangs large
bunches of plump grapes from silver Victorian stands.

But now it's time to say good-bye. My mom has sold her
house, and we make one last visit there to help her pack up
more than forty years of memories. We love the apartment
she has rented near my grandmother. She'll trade her yard
for a large balcony with a stunning view of the inland water-
way, where manatees and dolphins frequently swim by. She
has scored the best parking spot in the lot, directly next to the
building entrance. She's in a much better place now emotionally, having come to a settlement with my dad's partner, Jose,
who has agreed to buy my dad's share of the business. It means
that all those years he devoted to building his practice have
paid off for my mom. She'll be okay, and that's a huge relief to
all of us.

Beyoncé's "Diva" blasts from Emma's iPhone, which she
has plugged into a small speaker in one of the guest bedrooms.
It's the room where my mom has a huge dresser filled with
dress-up stuff. What started in my teen years as her collec-
tion of costume jewelry has morphed into a massive treasure
trove of fantasy: vintage decorative rhinestone tiaras, boas
in vibrant colors, beaded necklaces, fur collars and stoles,
leather and lace gloves, and sunglasses of all sizes from every

era. Emma wonders what my mom will do with it all; after all, none of it is a necessity, especially when you're downsizing from a roomy three-bedroom home to a compact two-bedroom apartment.

"Take all of it or none of it," Mom says, offering to ship it to New York for us. But Emma tells her it wouldn't be the same in our apartment. "The fun of dress-up is doing it here," she says affectionately, as she gently pinches her grandmother's cheek. In an anything-for-my-granddaughter moment, my mom says she will take it all to her new apartment and put it somewhere.

"I'd rather keep what makes you happy than have a couch," she says.

"Don't be dramatic, Sunshine!" Emma says. We all laugh and agree to sift through everything, choosing our very favorite items to keep. She'll give the rest to friends who have always admired her taste.

Emma pulls out two vintage rhinestone tiaras and then grabs the basket of oversize sunglasses. When we put them on, the combination of shades and tiaras makes us look like we're prepping to duck paparazzi. Or at least that's how we act as we stand in front of a large mirror and take dozens of selfies, each more outrageously posed than the previous one.

"The queen and her princess," my mom says, referring to her daughter and granddaughter. Emma corrects her: "You're the queen," she tells my mom. "This is the princess," she says, pointing to me. "And I'm the lady-in-waiting."

"What exactly are you waiting for?" my mom shoots back.

"A big kiss from you!" Emma responds with a wink. The girl is no dummy—she knows how to play her grandma.

If it's been a long time since you've played dress-up, let me tell you: there's nothing like a rhinestone tiara to lift your spirits and make you feel like royalty. Every girl should own one, whether it's store-bought or homemade. Whether you wear one or just place it somewhere as inspiration, it'll remind you that you are the queen of your life. Whatever you weigh, whatever your bank account balance, whether you feel loved or misunderstood, whether the stars are aligning and your dreams are coming true or you have to pick yourself up to start again, allow that headpiece to symbolize the power you possess. Do as Emma and I do: Put on a tiara, crank up the tunes, and dance like nobody's watching. It's a mood booster and a self-esteem enhancer disguised as a crown.

After our little tiara party, we spend an hour with Grandma Evelyn at her place. She knows who we are even if she can't remember our names, and her indomitable spirit is still there. When Peter asks if he can get her anything, thinking perhaps a glass of water, she replies bluntly, "Yes, a Whopper with fries." Peter and Jake head out to Burger King while Emma, my mom, Grandma, and I watch a *Golden Girls* marathon. That sitcom from the late eighties was one that she and I watched religiously during my youth. Her mind is clearly fading but not enough to stop her from laughing in all the right places, even if she's just mimicking us. My mom is sure that she's out of it, but I say if she can still laugh, then it's all good.

Evelyn's husband, my late grandpa Harvey, loved to say, "If the sun's shining, let's celebrate." Each morning when we get up, it means we're lucky to have another day here, especially since our time isn't guaranteed. Those are twenty-four hours for us to reign supreme. When you treat yourself royally—like a good and benevolent queen, not an effete let-them-eat-cake one—you'll see your power and confidence grow. You may not need a tiara to make it happen, but trust me, it helps. Put yours on from time to time, and rule your life.

Put on your tiara and dance.

LOVE AND SERVICE

Everybody can be great...because anybody can serve. You don't have to have a college degree to serve. You don't have to make your subject and verb agree to serve. You only need a heart full of grace. A soul generated by love.

—*Martin Luther King Jr.*

22

Give Back with a Quick Hand

When I felt stuck in a rut post-Shift, I knew I had to shake things up and get out of my own head. I needed to connect to something bigger than myself and put my own problems in perspective. I wanted to stop thinking about Tory and instead focus on helping others. I have always had an affinity for jumping into action during news-making crises because it has never felt right for me to sit back and do nothing. Every time I commit to helping, I feel good that I am able to reach out to the people who need it most. As my friend Dana reminds me, doing something for someone else pumps up your self-esteem in a more genuine way than getting a mani-pedi or changing your hairstyle. You'll forget what polish you chose on any given day but you'll always remember the coffee and blankets you gave the homeless woman to keep her warm, or the laughter of the kids in the library as they watched you act out their favorite fairytale.

After 2005's Hurricane Katrina, watching the devastation in New Orleans on TV, I think: *I've got to do something.* I know that helping people find jobs, especially when they've lost everything, will be critical in their long-term recovery. Peter thinks it's a bit extreme, but with contributions from family and friends, my brother, David, and I get on a flight to Houston. We head to the Astrodome, where many New Orleans residents have been bused. David envisions a possible documentary while I believe my background in helping women find jobs could come in handy. Inside the Astrodome I find a sea of broken people with no place to go. David starts shooting video and I hold up a handwritten posterboard sign that asks ARE YOU LOOKING FOR A JOB?

I'm approached by hundreds of people who've been evacuated. Most work minimum-wage jobs as janitors and housekeepers, fast-food line cooks, store clerks, waitresses, and dishwashers. I give advice and share what information I have at my fingertips. Certain drug chains, for example, will transfer jobs from their New Orleans stores to other cities. So will a number of major retail outlets. This is good news to many people there, and I'm glad to relay it.

Then I meet Doris. She's twenty-two and has been living in a New Orleans public housing project with her boyfriend, Michael, and their four-year-old son, Michael Jr. When the storm hits and the water rises above four feet, Doris puts her son in a plastic tub and floats him along to what she hopes is safety. At a highway overpass, she finds Michael's grandmother connecting with relatives for a drive to Alabama. Michael Jr. heads off with Grandma while Doris and Michael make their way to the convention center, the city's main evacuation point.

All hell is breaking loose there, a squalid mess of overflowing toilets and garbage strewn everywhere. Two days later, buses evacuate everyone to Houston's Astrodome.

Doris sleeps on an Army-issue cot there and learns that Michael Jr. has made it safely to Alabama. She had been working at a Taco Bell in New Orleans, and together we learn that the company will help her get a job in Houston at one of its locations. Driving around in a rental car, I help Doris find an apartment. I convince a building manager to accept her $541 public housing allotment for a condo that rents for considerably more. I fall in love with Doris and with the donated money I buy clothing and furniture to help her remake her life.

Doris knows true despair yet faces it fearlessly. It is far too simplistic to say that Doris is my reality check, a woman who reminds me that I am lucky to have my kind of problems and not hers. She loves big and encourages me to do the same, connecting me with my own heart. I'll always be in her corner. She can count on me for that.

But the truth is that other people can count on me, too. When I'm on your side, you get a cheerleader who wants you to win. I'm not the sexy-outfit-and-pom-poms type, but I'll devote my time to make great things happen for you. I'm proud of that and no one can take it away from me. When I fall in love with a product, I can't wait to put it on TV, which can change the trajectory of a business. When I like the people behind an item, I seek out magazine editors and store owners to get them more visibility and sales. When they succeed, I try to give them a spot on my event stages so they can share their challenges and triumphs with others. I don't do it because they beg or expect it, and I don't do it because I want anything in return. I help them because they *deserve* to be successful. They're good at what they do. They show up. They deliver, even when nobody's looking.

Eight years after Katrina, I meet Doris in New Orleans at a conference called FestiGals where I'm speaking. The women who are gathered here are the backbone of the city they have fought hard to bring back from the brink. The rest of the country might be ready to write off New Orleans as a lost cause, but not these women. From the dais, I point to Doris, who is standing with Peter in the back of the ballroom. I tell her story and how, after remaining in Houston for a year after the storm, she returned to the city she loved. She came back, I say, because New Orleans will always be her home. I can feel the emotion as the crowd stirs. The room begins to buzz, and within seconds everyone gets up from their seats, without any prompting from me, and gives Doris a prolonged standing ovation, the first time that's ever happened to her. Doris, who hasn't said a word, beams with tears in her eyes from the rear of the room.

Afterwards, women line up to shake Doris's hand and thank her for returning to New Orleans. They tell me they are grateful to me for coming to speak to them, and they talk about their city with deep affection and fierce pride. But then, nearly to a woman, they tell me their difficulties: finding work, losing weight, asking for a raise, and demanding the respect they think they deserve at home and on the job. Many say they are better at helping other people than they are at helping themselves. Self-esteem is a big issue.

Walking out of the hotel, I can't help wishing that more women felt as good about themselves as these women do about their city. I wish that, as women, we would fight for our own lives, health, careers, and happiness with the same unwavering love that we shower on our hometowns or sports teams. I wish more women in that room gave themselves a fraction of the love that they have given New Orleans.

Ever since they were young, I have taught our kids that the secret to living is giving. On a school holiday when they were eleven, Emma and Jake began holding bake sales in front of our apartment on Eighty-Sixth Street. It's something lots of kids do in small towns across America, but on the streets of Manhattan a kids' bake sale is an anomaly. Peter sets up a table with a red-checkered tablecloth where they arrange cookies, brownies, cakes, and lemonade to sell. It's a busy street and sidewalk, with many passersby heading to the subway at the corner. Amazingly, after just three hours, they have $300 in their till. One man is so amused to see kids doing a bake sale in Manhattan that he hands them a $50 bill for two brown-ies. "Keep the change," he says. Inspired by their success, they continue to hold Saturday morning bake sales and within a few weeks amass an astounding $1,000. Then the big question arises.

"What should we do with it?" Emma asks me.

"Let's save it," says Jake, who may still have the first dollar anyone ever gave him.

"How about we give it away?" I say.

With *Good Morning America* gearing up for its annual holi-day coat drive, I suggest we buy parkas for kids. After some back-and-forth about why we'd *give away* money that they earned, Emma and Jake endorse the idea of helping out other children. They get it. We all head to Conway, a discount store on West 116th Street. With some prodding, the manager sells us parkas for $10 apiece because she thinks the kids are cute and understands it's for a good cause. We stuff the car with one hundred coats. In a live segment later that week, *Good Morning America* newsreader Chris Cuomo asks Emma and Jake how they made all the money.

"Bake sales," Jake replies.

"That's a lot of money from bake sales," says Chris, ever skeptical.

"Even though they take the same effort to bake, we learned that you can charge a lot more for brownies than you can cookies," Emma shoots back truthfully, unfazed by his challenging question. "So we loaded up on brownies."

"Looks like you've learned a few of your mom's moneymaking skills," Chris says, convinced, high-fiving them both. That experience kicks off a love of giving for Jake and Emma, and they have cherished the opportunity to help others ever since.

Fast-forward to 2012. During Hurricane Sandy, I read an online post by pop icon Jon Bon Jovi. "We may not have electricity but we have power. This is what we do. We help others who are in need," he says after Sandy cuts a swath through the metropolitan area, uprooting thousands of homes, causing billions of dollars in damage, and crushing the spirits of many residents in New York, New Jersey, and Connecticut.

My life has not been affected at all by this storm: we are safe in our home, our electricity works, and our lives are unscathed. The kids still take the subway to school and other than a few downed tree limbs and other debris from the storm, Peter and I walk to work as if nothing has happened. Meanwhile tens of thousands of people just miles from us find themselves suddenly homeless or living in waterlogged homes, their lives turned inside out. When Peter goes to the stationery store a few doors down from our office, the owner is in tears because her business storage room on Staten Island has been swept away in the storm and her house next door badly damaged. He contributes to a fund set up to help her get back up and running. We get a taste of what it's like when friends across the Hudson River in New Jersey report that they lost their car in the storm and that their apartment has no electricity and probably won't for days. They ask us to care for their two large dogs. We do, and Marly is thrilled to have playmates.

Giving money to the Red Cross or any number of charity organizations to dispense is a perfectly fine option. But I wanted to give money directly to the people impacted by the storm. So I put together an online public crowdfunding campaign to show that ordinary people care and are not willing to place the lives of those who've been affected solely in the hands of government relief organizations and charities.

My goal is to raise $10,000 in ten days. I figure that if we spread the word on our websites, in mass emails, and through social media, that $1,000 a day will be a stretch but doable. Yet within hours of launching our campaign, I see that I've struck a chord—we're up to $5,000. Ten days later when the campaign ends, we've raised a whopping $100,000. That's when the excitement begins, because I know from experience that nothing feels as good as giving.

The storm has left Liz Kilborn, a young professional from Hoboken, New Jersey, with just the clothes on her back. She is stunned when I reach her at work. "Want to go shopping?" I ask this stranger, who initially thinks it's a prank call. When we meet at The Limited she's in tears, wearing donated Salvation

Army clothes with missing buttons. She tries on a bunch of tops and pants and I buy everything she likes. From there we carry our stuffed shopping bags to Nine West, where she picks out a pair of shoes, which she says is enough to last her for a bit. "No way," I say. "You need more than one pair," and we buy another. A few hours and a $1,000 wardrobe later, Liz is in tears as we say good-bye to each other. This time those tears are happy ones.

Every weekend during that November and into December, Peter, Emma, Jake, and I get into our trusty Honda Pilot and head to hard-hit Staten Island. The kids hardly view this as a chore. They want to accompany us. They were just seven when Katrina hit, and they don't remember anything about it. But now they're fourteen and they can't believe the stories they hear on TV. They both want to help. We center on Staten Island because Susie Rausch, a publicist I know from my PR days, sends an email saying that her house wasn't affected but many of her neighbors' lives are in turmoil. A few have lost all of their possessions. We set about buying things for residents Susie identified for us.

Ray Egers, a retired New York City firefighter, plans to rebuild his home himself if he can get power tools to replace the ones that were ruined when water from the Atlantic Ocean flooded his home. In anticipation of the coming renovation, he guts his entire waterlogged house right down to the studs to let everything dry out. We head to Home Depot with him to buy all the stuff he needs to get moving. Through her tears his wife, Maryann, shows us one of the few mementos that survived the devastating high tide, simply because it was hung high on a wall. It's a beautiful collage of family photos dating back years.

At Home Depot we also buy a washer and dryer for a stunned couple and a refrigerator and stove for a young mom. Then we go on a shopping spree at Target with a young family of four. They are all beyond grateful.

The highlight of our time on Staten Island is a holiday party at Public School 41, just blocks from many of the affected homes. Susie, working with the school, makes sure that 115 families who have been hardest hit show up for the breakfast. They think they're about to choose one toy per family from the Toys for Tots initiative that is set up. But when the breakfast ends, a school administrator introduces me and says that I have a little gift for each of them. As they walk from the cafeteria, I hand each family a $500 Visa gift card so they can buy presents or necessities for themselves. The tears flow.

As planned, in a matter of weeks I give away the entire $100,000 we have raised to families on Staten Island and in New Jersey. I have never felt better during any holiday season, before or since. I've stayed in touch with the families, and for the one-year anniversary of Sandy, the Egerses sent me a dish that sits on my dresser. I have looked at it more than a few times when I'm blue, and each time it lifts my spirits. Painted on it is a quote from Eleanor Roosevelt: "Many people will walk in and out of your life, but only true friends will leave footprints in your heart." The Egerses probably don't realize it, but they and the other strong, resilient people I met after Sandy did far more for me than I did for them.

You don't have to raise $100,000 to make a difference, nor do you need to wait for catastrophic events to happen in order to lend a hand. Begin small, right near home. Perhaps you have an elderly neighbor who needs help getting to and from the grocery store or would love for you to pop in once a week with your iPhone so she can FaceTime with her grandchildren in another state. A nearby homeless shelter or soup kitchen—or one run by a church in your area—is likely in need of volunteers or contributions of cash and product year-round. Sign up for a fund-raising walk for a cause you care about or ask how you can best support that organization. If you love books, offer to read to kids in a classroom or consider giving a hand to the local library. There's no shortage of ways to help.

Even a simple act of kindness can change someone's entire life.

23

Make a Difference
with a Lasting Heart

Reaching out to others doesn't only mean organizing a grandiose fund-raiser or marshaling the troops to respond to tragedy. It can mean dropping off some food to your neighbors who had twins and are feeling understandably overwhelmed. It can mean sending a text to someone just to say you're thinking of her. It simply means hearts touching hearts, which reminds us that we're all connected on some deeper level.

We experience that human bond the first Sunday of every November, when more than fifty thousand runners and many more supporters end the iconic New York City Marathon in our backyard on the Upper West Side. Emma and I walk around to see runners huddled under their shiny silver heat-shield capes as they look for friends and family. Everyone is in a festive mood, even though it's cold and blustery as the sun begins to set after the race. We join the throngs of people who walk up to random runners, perfect strangers, many from different countries.

"Congrats, you did it!" says Emma, never one to talk to anyone she doesn't know. "Hey, good for you! Proud of you!" she says to a woman runner who is looking for someone she planned to meet in front of Starbucks on Columbus Avenue. *"Merci,"* the French woman says shyly.

I love the sense of camaraderie and community that happens as thousands of people from all walks of life and different parts of the world gather here for this big event. During the race, fans cheer for people they know first and foremost: "Go, Marcia!" "Kill it, Francine!" "You got this, Josie!" (We still use the plastic orange cups from the party we threw for my brother when he ran the Marathon in 2009, the ones that say DAVID DID IT!) But they also scream out support to all runners. Even people like us who rarely go to all sorts of sporting events find themselves moved by the marathon.

It taps into a spirit that lies just beneath the surface of many New York City residents, one that was most poignantly displayed to the world when the Twin Towers came crashing down, killing close to three thousand people. Emma and Jake had started preschool the day the planes hit. I remember holding their hands the next day when we took a cooked ham and turkey to the firehouse on West Eighty-Third Street, just blocks from our apartment. The fireman who greeted us had a stunned look on his face because 343 fellow firemen and paramedics had died in the attacks.

The Marathon, the biggest city event of the year, has nothing to do with team pride, loyalty to city, or even physical fitness. It's about human endurance and potential: pushing beyond what we once believed impossible and aiming to achieve a personal best, driven by fortitude that can't be cowed by brutal winds, miles to go, or pure exhaustion. The on-their-sleeve emotion and warmth of the moment lasts for several hours as the runners cross the finish line. Late that night I scroll through Instagram posts from the race, and the best are photos of the signs that lined the runners' path:

IN YOUR MIND YOU'RE A KENYAN.

THIS SEEMS LIKE AN AWFUL LOT OF WORK FOR A FREE BANANA.

MY PACE OR YOURS.

YOU'RE RUNNING BETTER THAN OUR GOVERNMENT.

WHEN YOU ARE GOING THRU HELL KEEP GOING.

PAIN IS TEMPORARY. INTERNET RACE RESULTS ARE FOREVER.

For days, I am buoyed by the energy and drive on display by people who commit to running 26.2 miles and then actually do it. It's a powerful reminder to me that no matter how big my challenge, no matter how audacious my dream, I can accomplish great things the way marathoners do: one step at a time.

A few weeks later, on Thanksgiving night, ABC airs Robin Roberts' *Thank You, America*, a celebration of America's unsung heroes. I'm in tears when a dad from St. Cloud, Minnesota, explains why he and his wife are foster parents. "Someone has to step up and open their hearts to these kids." I am so moved by the broadcast that I decide to kick off a holiday crowdfunding campaign, which I call Strangers Helping Strangers.

I know that contributions to my latest campaign will never reach anything near Sandy levels, because there's no clear crisis or emergency. But we don't need a storm to spread good cheer, I tell potential supporters. "The Marathon reminds us that any time is a good time to cheer for people who need it. Bringing a smile to someone's face should be something we do every single day."

I'm astounded when Strangers Helping Strangers raises a whopping $50,000, far more than I ever expected. For weeks I've been inspired by reading Neediest Cases stories, an annual fund-raiser in the *New York Times*. I find a story about Taylor Turntime, a nineteen-year-old girl who has been in and out of foster care since she was four, particularly poignant. With a ton of willpower and against all odds, she is now one of the three percent—*three percent*—of foster kids who have made it to college. But first, she needs a dress for her high school prom. Neediest Cases comes through with a $100 Marshalls gift card that she uses to buys a strapless, peach floor-length gown.

"I had the best dress at prom," Taylor tells the *Times*. "I felt like a princess."

That floors me and I decide that I must meet this young woman. I track down Fabienne Pierre, Taylor's mentor at the Children's Aid Society who is mentioned in the *Times* piece, and ask her what is on Taylor's Christmas wish list. "She never celebrated Christmas so getting her to dream big and find out what she wanted was a bit hard," Fabienne tells me in an email. "She's also so humble and independent that it was a bit hard for her to actually think about something."

Nonetheless, Taylor comes through with her wish list, and this girl thinks big: She'd like to take a trip to South Africa and Ghana because she's passionate about African-American culture. She dreams of touching big turtles in Kiholo Bay in Hawaii and meeting President Obama. I'm in no position to deliver those things, but her wish for a dorm room makeover catches my eye. "I'd love to just walk into my room and feel like I walked in a castle," Taylor writes.

Fabienne says that another youth, Maurice Reid, a student

at New York University, has recently aged out of the foster care system. He is struggling to make ends meet on his own. He has taken out a student loan and works part-time to help pay the remaining balance for school and to support himself. He's a member of Phi Theta Kappa Honor Society, on the New Yorkers for Children Youth Advisory Board, and participates in several community service projects. Like Taylor, his Christmas wish list is to spruce up his room with a new rug, lamp, and comforter.

I decide that I've got to meet Maurice, too. With Fabienne's help, we agree to all meet at the Target store in Harlem. Neither Taylor nor Maurice has any idea why we're meeting there. When they press Fabienne about it, she says that a woman wants to buy one item for each of their bedrooms. They are thrilled with that, Fabienne tells me.

"One item?" I say when I meet Taylor and Maurice. "Oh no. We're doing *total room makeovers*." Fabienne laughs and Maurice and Taylor are visibly stunned. Needless to say, they're blown away by the surprise and are kids in a candy shop for the next few hours. Like cautious buyers at a high-end auction, they examine every item very carefully, and soon their shopping carts overflow with pillows, sheets, comforters, small rugs, pictures, and mirrors.

My assistant, Gianna, is with me and we all have fun snapping photos of their haul to post on social media. We want contributors to our campaign to be able to see some of the deserving people they've directly helped. It's a joyous experience for everyone. Gianna and I agree that it's the longest time either of us has ever spent in a Target—and the most meaningful, too. We marvel at how meticulous Taylor and Maurice are about their choices, making sure they not only need each item but that it's something they really value. Getting it all just right is important to them. A

few weeks later when they're back at school, both send me photos and guided video tours of their new dorm rooms. "It's good to
know that someone out there is thinking about us and wants us
to succeed and be happy," Maurice writes in an email.

Fabienne also tells me about a third youth, named Angelique
Salizan, who spent sixteen years, virtually her entire life, in the
foster care system. Now a freshman at Binghamton University
in upstate New York, she has a perfect 4.0 grade point average.
She is spending her holiday break in New York City, working an
overnight shift at McDonald's to make a few bucks. She hopes
to become a nurse therapist so she can help soldiers returning
from active duty in war zones. Her Christmas wish list includes
an iPad mini, Barnes & Noble gift card, and makeup. Imagine
Angelique's surprise when Gianna and I walk up to her unan-
nounced at a Starbucks. She has no idea what this is about or
who we are as we hand her every single thing on her wish list.

A week later, Peter and I are headed back to Target with an
even bigger shopping list. Fabienne has connected me with her
peers at The Children's Village, a foster care facility in Westchester. We're on a mission to buy basketball socks, board games,
and other small stuff for fifty boys there. "I can assure you that
whatever you give them they can use and will genuinely appreciate," says Amy DelliPaoli, a warm, caring woman who runs the
volunteer services there. "They're not used to getting gifts."

On a snowy day before Christmas, with fifty holiday tote bags
brimming with goodies, Peter and I drive north on the Henry
Hudson Parkway past the George Washington Bridge toward
The Children's Village in Dobbs Ferry. It's our first time there
and we don't know what to expect. "It looks like a little college,"
Peter says as we drive into the 180-acre campus dotted with

small brick and cinderblock cottages, administration offices, and classrooms.

To one degree or another, all the boys at The Children's Village have heartbreaking stories. Maybe it's a brush with the law that lands them here or a previous foster home that didn't work out for any number of reasons. Some have been abandoned by parents or guardians who are in prison, rehab, or in the throes of drug or alcohol addiction. Many have no known relatives to care for them, or if they do, those relatives are in no position—or have no desire—to take them in. It's the dark underbelly of civilization that is largely hidden from the rest of us, one that these kids are mostly born into through no fault of their own. It's no wonder that so many of the boys struggle with psychological issues.

I remember the man from Minnesota in Robin Roberts' Thanksgiving special on ABC: "Someone has to step up and open their hearts to these kids." The Children's Village does that. Although every kid is awaiting placement in a foster home, the truth is that some will never find families willing to take them in. They'll end up spending their entire childhood at the Village, which was built on a farm purchased by the New York Juvenile Asylum in the early 1900s. "Orphans who were placed here helped build the campus, brick by brick," Amy says as we walk together to the first cottage. The group homes are comfortable but definitely have an institutional feel: linoleum floors are clean and buffed and signs encourage everyone to be polite and kind, to respect each other. We walk into the living rooms of each cottage to find six to ten boys doing what most kids their age do: listening to music on MP3s, playing video games, or watching TV.

I decide before we arrive that I'll just jump right in, figuring the boys won't take to a woman who displays a lack of confidence. It's always worked well for me before: people respect confidence far more than they do shyness. "Hi guys," I say as we walk through the door. "Thought I'd stop by just to say hello and bring you a little Christmas cheer."

A few kids stare at me, sullen, silent, and brooding. Others don't look up from their video games. But one by one kids approach us, and with a little prodding, Peter and I engage them in light banter. We're both amazed at how hungry they are for attention. With encouragement they chat about video games, the dinner menu, and basketball. They're just kids. I can tell that the video games they're playing are old, so I ask if they'd like some new ones. I suggest that they figure out as a group what new game they'd really like and I will send it after the holidays. But several boys immediately shout out in unison: "*Call of Duty.* We want *Call of Duty.*" I know nothing about video games, but enough to recognize that's a violent game. Instead of rejecting their request out of hand, I think quickly about what game Jake plays at home: "How about *Madden*?" That gets a thumbs-up. I can't be all bad if I know the hottest football game for Xbox.

In the other houses, in addition to choosing a video game, I ask the boys what book they'd love to have, any title or subject they want. A few kids, but not many, make suggestions on the spot, such as the biography of Miami Heat star Dwayne Wade, *The Guinness Book of World Records*, and anything by Bill Nye the Science Guy. I send books a few weeks later. On our way to the next cottage, I wonder out loud if our teeny kindness means anything to kids with such vast needs. "I can see them thinking, 'too little, too late.'" Amy assures me that any and all gestures count with these kids, whether they show it or not. "Many of these boys have no one."

I am struck by their innocence and wonder how spending their childhood years in a group home will affect them. Thank God for The Children's Village. It's an institution, but clearly the staff cares for every kid and invites in people like us to follow their lead. If you have a heart, they say, you have all the equipment you need to give. It's as simple as that.

Amy encourages us to come back. "No need to bring gifts. The gift is your time." She says that just talking means more to them than any material stuff. They aren't used to many visitors, so she says we did well by keeping the conversation flowing even in the face of some nonresponsive kids. "To see someone besides the staff care about them is big," Amy says. The Children's Village is always looking for mentors, she says, and most of the kids would benefit from a trip to a diner since they have never held a menu or interacted with a waiter or been given much of a choice about what to eat. This is sophisticated Westchester, fifteen miles from the heart of Manhattan, the epicenter of cutting-edge business, science, and education. And yet here are kids without permanent homes or families, just wanting what all of us want, which is to be loved. It's heartbreaking.

On the drive home, Peter and I decide we want to be more involved. We head back to Dobbs Ferry one Saturday to take a daylong mentor training program and submit paperwork for background checks, fingerprinting, and evaluations to become mentors. We will be assigned a kid, likely a boy about twelve years old, and visit with him regularly for the next year. As we get to know him and his interests, Amy says, our plans will develop: dinners off campus, museums, ball games, or just walks in a park. During training we learn there's nothing wrong with doing basic things such as simple errands that families do every day. There's value in a kid seeing everyday normal life, we're told.

I'm drawn to mentoring a foster kid because for once in my life it's not a one-and-done kind of thing, like a fund-raiser. It's a long-term commitment. Peter and I have spent the past twenty years nurturing our kids together, and we think we're good at guiding young people. We're ready as a couple to share what we've learned and to open ourselves to new lessons from the kids we meet.

In some ways, our character is judged by how well we treat those who can do nothing for us in return. Few things feel as good as giving. "I've learned that you shouldn't go through life with a catcher's mitt on both hands; you need to be able to throw something back," Maya Angelou said. We assume we don't have time, but we can make time for what matters. Some activities zap us of energy while others restore our energy tenfold. Giving is one of those things. Do yourself a favor: recharge yourself by committing to doing something for others that'll make you feel really good about yourself. There are lots of ways to give back, and most of them do not involve money. Our time is extraordinarily valuable—to us and to those who can benefit from it. Volunteer to be a Big Sister. Register to read to children in an inner-city classroom. Visit a nursing home and provide company to a resident who doesn't have family nearby. Socialize with animals in a shelter. Part of me has always been a big giver for selfish reasons: it makes me feel good inside. I continue not only because the world needs my help, but also because *I* need the feeling of joy that overflows from my heart when I do it.

Few things feel as good as giving.

24

Help Someone Fulfill a Dream

Emma is all about pop culture. The Latest Thing fascinates her. Peter marvels at how she can expertly lip-sync lyrics to songs that he swears must be in another language. They go back and forth about it regularly, with him saying that in his day, before there was indoor plumbing and electricity or airplanes, at least you could understand the lyrics. "Feeling old, are you, Daddy?" Emma asks.

Our girl is also a fashionista who spends hours checking out the newest clothes, jewelry, and accessories online and in magazines. No detail escapes her attention. For the past few years, unprompted, Emma has given me many ideas of hot brands to consider for my "Deals & Steals" segments. More than a few of them wind up on-air and she never fails to ask how certain items sold, especially the ones she recommended.

When she asks about a popular jewelry line that she had suggested and I had then featured on *Good Morning America*, I tell her that they made hundreds of thousands of dollars in sales. Her eyes widen in amazement.

"I should have a jewelry business," she says.

"So start one," I tell her.

I've always thought that Emma had all the markings of a Mini Me. She is strong and decisive with a good BS detector, useful qualities when you own a small business. But I also know that while her grades are good, her SATs are nothing to brag about. She needs something that will make her high school years pop on college applications. Starting a jewelry business and getting it up and running while balancing homework and other activities can't hurt. To my surprise, Emma takes my challenge and runs with it. I say "to my surprise" not because I think she is lazy, but because between their social lives and academic demands, high school students have a full load. Running any business takes time and commitment.

Her initial concept is in homage to my dad, who was a sharp dresser. She repurposes his colorful striped cotton shirts and bold-patterned silk ties by cutting them into wrist-wrap bracelets featuring small charms. When she posts photos on Instagram, friends ask where she bought them. Orders for her wrist ties start to come in as girls read Emma's story about why she made them: to honor her grandfather's impeccable taste in clothing by recycling his wardrobe into bracelets.

With that initial success she creates a brand, Em John Jewelry, based on a nickname that stuck at her summer sleep-away camp. She goes online and learns how to build her own website and figures out how to set up and accept payments via PayPal. She designs business cards and packaging inserts by herself using Vistaprint, and weighs what works and what doesn't as she goes along. She's the only girl, perhaps the only student, in her three-hundred-strong senior class who runs her own business.

A lot of it is hit-and-miss for Emma—as it is with many entrepreneurs. She soon learns that while silk tie strips are colorful and unique, they're also a hassle because they don't stay on wrists very well, especially for active teenage girls who remove them for showers, swimming, or sweaty gym work-outs. So Emma begins to design fun bracelets featuring rubber beads. She finds a manufacturer who accepts low minimum wholesale orders of her custom-designed Lucite charms, which replace the original metal ones. Some sell well, some not at all, but nothing seems to derail her enthusiasm. That's an early sign to me that she's got what it takes to make it as a business owner. Her excitement is infectious and keeps me pumped to stay focused on my own business initiatives, which have been progressing nicely of late.

Emma and I have both traveled far in a short period of time. While maintaining her grades and juggling all the teen-age social stuff that comes with high school, she has also cre-ated something from nothing. She now has a business that is catching on and that has taught her many elements of entrepre-neurship at a young age.

I awaken one Saturday morning to find her nervously toss-ing jewelry samples on her bed. She is anxious because this is her very first trunk show; it's at Olive and Bette's, an upscale women's clothing store with four locations in New York. "I'm not sure how many pieces I should bring," she says, close to tears. "I'm terrified that no one is going to buy anything and I'm going to be standing there like a loser all day. I'm freaking out that none of the friends who promised me they'd show up will actually come."

In an instant, whatever challenges I have in my life give way to motherly concern for my girl. I realize that nothing is more important than instilling in her the confidence she'll need if she ever hopes to have a successful enterprise. Even though I'd feel just as vulnerable in her shoes, I have to be strong for her. "Set the bar low," I tell her. "This is a learning experience, a chance to see what a trunk show is like, to meet with potential customers, to get a taste of the retail world. Today it's not about sales but about giving the impression to people that you're excited to share your designs, that you can handle yourself, and that you're committed."

That seems to work, and helping her focus on her issues allows me to backburner any of my own worries for a while. For her big retail debut, Emma selects a cute cotton dress, sneakers, and a well-worn jean jacket. I tell her she looks great, which she does. An hour later, Emma stands at her small table near the front entrance to the store as women come and go. Some stop to look at the bracelets while others completely ignore her. But Emma's pre-show jitters have worn off and I can see that she is comfortable and confident. Either that or she is putting on a very brave face.

Within a matter of minutes a teenage girl whispers to her mom that she'd like to try on a bracelet. "Hey! How are you?" Emma asks without any prompting from me. She launches into the story of how and why she started her business. The mom buys her daughter two, one for her and one for her camp friend. They leave after handing the front-desk cashier $28, half of which will go to Emma. You'd have thought she'd won millions at Powerball, such is my girl's glee.

"Your first trunk show sale!" I say, high-fiving her as she does a little jig while looking around in hopes of not being caught by the sales associates. As the day progresses, Emma's friends show up to support her and they all buy bracelets, a welcome sign of female solidarity for which Emma is extremely grateful. Emma will soon write about this day for her college essay, with an optimism that shines through. While I have been working diligently for months to reassess what matters to me, my daughter, with some gentle encouragement, sees more stars in the sky. I couldn't be happier.

Within a few months her Em John Jewelry business is smoking. She has expanded from bracelets to zippered pouches featuring inspirational messages like WE ALL HAVE THE SAME NUMBER OF HOURS IN A DAY AS BEYONCÉ. She fills online wholesale and retail orders each week.

"Another day, another K for me, another day, another A for you," she teases Jake, using the slang for "one thousand."

When he was young, Jake was fascinated with money. During one comical scene when he was six, he demanded that a Chase bank officer show him the vault where she told him she would put the $100 I'd given him to start a savings account. After failing to talk him out of it, she took him by the hand and walked him into the vault. Only then did Jake agree to part with his money. Now a perfect GPA is the number that drives him.

But money motivates Emma—and not in a greedy way. Without any prompting from Peter or me, her goal is to make enough to pay for her first year of college, and she's on her way.

Things work out when you put effort into them, and Emma's business is a case in point. There's a distinction between sitting back and hoping or praying that things will work out and giving your all to make them happen.

By helping Emma grow Em John, I am rediscovering the joy of creating. She has turned our dining room table into an after-school workshop. It's usually piled high with colored rubber beads, charms of assorted shapes and styles, jump rings, plastic packaging, business cards, and shipping envelopes. She enlists all of us to help her assemble pieces, but this is her vision and hers alone. She decides how to coordinate colors like a silver heart on turquoise beads or a clear emoji with purple beads. I watch her popularity grow as she connects with bloggers and the Instagram crowd, offering to send product samples in exchange for posts. Her batting average is impressive: almost everyone she reaches out to responds and says that they like her story. It's hard not to root for a high school entrepreneur who's hustling.

Soon Emma hits the mother lode: her bracelets are featured in *Oprah* magazine, a dream for anyone who sells a product. Emma knows that appearing in *O* is a really big deal, but she is not prepared for the avalanche of orders that comes in as a result. Several stores place wholesale orders, and she trades her backpack for a shopping bag filled with packages that she dutifully ships from the post office each day after school.

There's great joy in helping someone fulfill a dream, as I've tried to do with Emma. I begin to understand that I can feel as much joy for someone else's successes as I can my own. I'm inspired by all that she's doing, and her infectious enthusiasm has reignited my own creative spark. For months while I was living in my funky fog, I felt as though I'd lost that spark. I'd force myself to write, only to stare at a blank page. I'd hit DELETE over and over because the words just weren't right. I'd try to be clever, but all my ideas fell flat.

Then I just stopped trying so hard. I stopped trying to be creative and focused instead on being content. Slowly my creativity reemerged. That her success provided this valuable reverse mentoring for me is a huge bonus. Making something from nothing—whether it's a cake, a garden, or a scrapbook; a piece of jewelry or something from Play-Doh—is both fun and rewarding. Whatever it is, there's something deeply satisfying about using your hands, head, and heart. Think of ways to tap your creativity, either by helping others pursue their dream or by diving into a hobby you've often considered but put off. Both can give value that you may come to appreciate very soon.

When you give it your all, there's always a way.

25

Get a Pet

Some of the best things in life are right in front of us, but sometimes we don't notice them or we take them for granted. I am guilty of that when it comes to our beloved hound, Marly. He joined our family one weekend eight years ago when Peter pointed to a classified ad for pups in a local paper.

"Who wants to get a dog today?" he asked, as Emma and Jake went predictably wild, being ten at the time.

"We do!" they said. "Right now!" That settled that.

We had talked about getting a dog and I had always wanted a beagle, but I never thought we'd move so fast. Two hours later, we had an adorable beagle pup. Peter picked him from the litter because he was the best-looking one and stayed in the back of the cage while all the other pups jumped up to greet us. He liked the fact that Marly was more reserved and laid-back than his siblings.

Since that day Marly has primarily stuck to Peter, who walks, feeds, and pets him more than anyone else. But everyone in our house loves The Baby, which is what we call him.

Jake roughhouses with him after school, and Emma does homework on her bed with Marly at her feet. Each night after dinner, without fail, he jumps up on my side of the bed to keep me company while I work on my laptop. It's our special time together as he looks lovingly at me with his big brown eyes and I look right back while I rub his neck, which makes him go into something of a trance. I've always found it relaxing, too, but I never attached any real significance to our nightly ritual.

Then I read in the *New York Times* that a study by Japanese researchers found that dogs who gaze at their owners have elevated levels of oxytocin. That's a hormone in the brain associated with nurturing and attachment, similar to the feel-good feedback that bolsters bonding between parent and child. But the interesting part is that the researchers discovered that after receiving those long gazes from their pooches, the owners' levels of oxytocin increased, too. Who knew?

"A dog is the only thing on earth that loves you more than he loves himself," humorist Josh Billings said. The late *60 Minutes* pundit Andy Rooney wrote, "The average dog is a nicer person than the average person." And French leader Charles de Gaulle once said, "The better I get to know men, the more I find myself loving dogs." Ha! I still love people above all, but pets help us to be better versions of ourselves.

It wasn't until we almost lost him that I genuinely appreciated just how much Marly means to me. One night Peter lets him off the leash in Central Park to play with other dogs. He does it all the time, but for some reason this time Marly gets confused and they become separated. Within minutes, every dog owner is screaming Marly's name to help Peter locate him. Peter calls home in a panic to summon Jake, Emma, and me to the park to join in the search. The three of us race down our stairwell, which is faster than waiting for the elevator, only to find Marly waiting for us in the lobby. He is howling and his tail is wagging furiously with excitement. He had run more than a mile through the park and across dark, busy New York City streets to our building. The doorman says he scratched the front door just moments earlier to be let in. We had feared the worst and are all relieved and extremely impressed that he made his way back safely.

I never feed him and I rarely walk him. But I know I am witnessing pure love when Marly pushes my computer away with his nose and puts his head on my lap, waiting to be petted. I love this dog so much and he gives it back to me, even though the only thing I ever do for him is cuddle each and every night. Studies have found that dog owners are less likely to suffer from depression than those without pets. People with dogs have lower blood pressure in stressful situations than those without pets. One study even found that when people with borderline hypertension adopted dogs from a shelter, their blood pressure declined significantly within five months. Playing with a dog or cat can elevate levels of serotonin and dopamine, which calm and relax. Pet owners have lower triglyceride and cholesterol levels, both indicators of heart disease, than those without pets. Heart attack patients with dogs survive longer than those without. Pet owners over age sixty-five make thirty percent fewer visits to their doctors than those without pets.

What's more, numerous studies have linked dog ownership to weight loss: one study found that walking an overweight dog helped both the animal and its owner lose weight. Researchers also discovered that the dogs provide support in the same way as a human exercise buddy, but with greater consistency and no negative influence. Public housing residents who walked therapy dogs for up to twenty minutes, five days a week, lost an average of just over fourteen pounds in a year, without changing their diets. Another study found that people who got a dog walked thirty minutes more a week than they did before. One study after another points to exactly why a dog is a woman's best friend.

There's no shortage of research that touts the serious benefits of pet ownership. The bottom line is that having a dog can make life less anxious and stressful, add structure and exercise to your day, provide companionship, and help you start and maintain new friendships when you meet other dog owners.

When her beagle, Cookie, died at age fourteen, life coach Martha Beck blogged about losing a pet who had never left her side. In return, she says she got dozens of "emails, cards, letters and other varieties of kind wishes, just because my fat old dog died."

Thanking those who reached out to her, she wrote: "So many people have offered me love in the past few days, for no earthly reason except pure kindness, that I've come to a radical conclusion. It seems that the world is filled not only with human beings, but also with human beagles. People who love you even when you're not 'productive.' People who don't care how much you earn, sleep, weigh or vacuum. People who accept and encourage and care, even when you fall off the communication map for months on end. I'll never deserve to have you in my life, just as I never deserved to have Cookie. The miracle is we get love whether we deserve it or not. In fact, it may come to find us just when we think we deserve it least."

I know a pet is a huge responsibility and expense. For our family and millions like us, we wouldn't trade it for anything. If you don't already own one, consider the benefits of bringing home a pooch and getting unconditional love in return. If you're unsure about owning a pet, or if you live in a place that doesn't allow you to, think about offering to walk a neighbor's dog, pet-sit for a colleague who's going on vacation, volunteer a few times a month at your local animal shelter, or just pause to pet other people's dogs you meet in the park.

A pet can help you become a more loving version of yourself.

SHIFTING FOR GOOD

Instead of wondering when your next vacation is, maybe you should set up a life you don't need to escape from.

—*Seth Godin*

26

My New Shift Takes Hold

Some great news: Emma has been accepted to Boston University and Jake is committing to Tufts in nearby Medford. When they head to college in the fall, they will be only eight miles from each other, which is perfect for them and ideal for us when we visit. I take comfort in knowing they're headed *to* great things, not running *from* a home and a childhood that they're eager to flee. I know I'll be a puddle of tears when the day finally arrives, but right now I feel really excited about sending them off. My enthusiasm has little to do with a text my friend Shannon, the wife of a minister, sends when I share the news on Facebook. "Now you and Peter can have sex in any room anytime," she writes, adding several laughing-face emojis.

I'm happy for my kids because I'm in a good place.

The mysterious pain in my lower jaw that has dogged me for months in the hours right after I wake up has completely disappeared. So has a small, persistent rash on the right side of my face, which during the same time frame ran from just above my eye to underneath my ear. Antibiotics and two expensive prescription-strength creams from a dermatologist six months ago did not help, so I stopped seeing her and eventually gave up on finding a cure. Instead, I used makeup and did my best to cover the teeny red bumps and irritated skin.

Grabbing coffee together, David instantly notices that the rash is gone. "You're glowing," he says.

"Yeah, I'm not sure how it happened, but somehow that entire rash vanished on its own," I tell him.

Without hesitation, he scoffs at that notion. "The reason that rash went away has everything to do with your attitude." He seems somewhat bothered by what he perceives to be my naiveté, like *duh*.

I roll my eyes, which annoys him more, something an older sister can get away with.

"Don't you see it?" he asks, prepared to answer his own question. "Teeth grinding and skin rashes don't happen in a vacuum. They're symptoms of something happening in your body. It's your body's cry for help."

Hmmm, I think, this is interesting. I motion for him to continue.

"No more jaw pain and troubled skin are rewards from your body because you've been practicing calm each day for a prolonged period," he tells me with a seriousness that's developed from a passion project of his that's taken on new meaning. David has morphed into a student of stress management. This is the same adorable brother-expert who, during my first Shift, convinced me to buy all kinds of very expensive workout equipment because, he said, he knew what was best. I ended up chucking it all out with the exception of the treadmill in our bedroom.

But this is different. David is making a documentary on Dr. John Sarno, a controversial expert on chronic back pain. Sarno attributes a lot of pain—especially back pain—to underlying stress. His famous acolyte patients swear by him. People like Howard Stern and Larry David, both of whom my brother interviewed for his film, say Sarno turned their lives around. But Sarno is controversial because, unlike many physicians who prefer to operate on slipped discs and other back ailments, he urges patients to think about the underlying emotional causes of their pain, even when the pain is so intense they can barely move. He wants them to explore the reasons why they're so tightly wound.

More often than not, when they think about it, when they dive deep into the causes and make important lifestyle changes, it's bye-bye back pain. That's what David's telling me.

"You are now experiencing the genuine benefit that comes from acupuncture, meditation, moving more, giving back regularly, and calming the hell down," Dr. Dave says. "Before you got into all of that, your thoughts were so tightly wound that your body was paying the price."

I stare at him, but this time it's not in disbelief. I actually think my sweet little brother, all six-foot-two-inches of him, is absolutely right.

"That'll be three hundred dollars, please," he says, appreciating how impressed I am with his take on things. We both laugh, but it's no joke. I have consciously chosen to replace my hectic, frenzied pace with more moments where I take time to just breathe and smell the roses. He hands me his iPhone to watch an adorable video of Charlotte and Morgan, my three-year-old niece and one-year-old nephew, jumping on his bed. It ends with both kids collapsing in my sister-in-law Julie's arms as the three of them laugh, carefree, for another thirty seconds. David and I are now smiling, too, finding joy in the stuff that really matters. It is a daily conscious effort on my part. I have shed ongoing anxiety, regret about the past, and worry about the future by making a conscious effort to just be content and live in the moment.

Allow calm and joy to replace fear and anxiety.

Owning My Confidence

27

When I first Shifted, I laid out a specific road map for myself that was pretty straightforward: I needed to be disciplined about what and when I ate. I needed to take a hard look each morning at the number on the scale. And I needed to get up off my butt and move a lot more.

Shifting for Good has been much more of zigzag journey. The inner work of staying present, finding peace, feeling more joy, and sharing myself with the people I love has evolved over time. I was determined not to fall back into my old habits, not to succumb to the *poor me*s or the *if only*s that really never did me any good anyway. So I took steps that worked for me—the ones I've shared on these pages. Maybe it's because I am getting older or maybe it's because of the work I've done over the course of my journey, but now I really get it: Life isn't a dress rehearsal; it's our only shot, so we might as well get it right.

I learned some other lessons. For starters, being true to myself is essential. I'm glad I listened to Robin Roberts, whose mom taught her to make "her mess her message." I did that

197

when I finally shared my struggles with weight and reaped tremendous rewards: new friends, a loyal following of women who struggle like I have, and the satisfaction that comes from helping others overcome the same challenges.

I learned that there's internal and external power to sharing a weakness as long as you're honest about it. As Brené Brown, a popular American scholar who researches vulnerability and courage, says, "Owning our story can be hard but not nearly as difficult as spending our lives running from it. Embracing our vulnerabilities is risky but not nearly as dangerous as giving up on love and belonging and joy—the experiences that make us the most vulnerable. Only when we are brave enough to explore the darkness will we discover the infinite power of our light."

I also learned that feeling good takes work, just as relationships take work. It's been more than twenty years since my grandma advised me on marriage, and I think about her words often: "Marriage takes work; put yourself in charge of the household finances; and never take Peter for granted." But just as a good marriage takes work, so does a commitment to contentment. Unlike an annual vacation to relax and recharge, contentment must be part of a daily routine—a regular focus, not an occasional blip.

"People often say that motivation doesn't last. Well, neither does bathing—that's why we recommend it daily," said the late motivational speaker Zig Ziglar. In *The Shift*, I wrote that a key step of Shifting is having daily accountability: it's so easy to lose track of time and progress, but when you work on it daily, it becomes part of you and defines who you are. It becomes as natural as remembering to have a cup of coffee, as Bob Roth taught me about TM.

Remember, too, that it's important to enjoy the journey, not just the destination. Sometimes we're so obsessed with getting where we're headed that we don't savor the ride. Maybe it's because of the way we approached the road trips we've taken as a family, but never once did I hear a voice coming from the backseat, asking the question "Are we there yet?" It's always a good idea to make the ride as fun as the destination, otherwise you're apt to get bored, restless, or discouraged and give up too soon. That's why we belt out songs blasting on the radio whenever we go on road trips. Last year on the way to Florida we listened to the *Serial* podcast from National Public Radio and obsessed about Adnan Syed's guilt or innocence. We play games, tell jokes, share stories, and fantasize about our dreams on car rides. To avoid fast-food joints, we Yelp places along the way to find the best local restaurants. On Johnson family vacations, the rides are always as fun as the places we visit.

After my first Shift, I became too hooked on celebrating my weight loss and the reaction to the book. So much so that once that was over, I felt like I had nothing. I didn't know quite how to define myself. I had been The Fat Girl all my life and now that I wasn't, what was I exactly? So as I began the journey toward Shifting for Good, I vowed I would greet each day as it presented itself, noticing my joys and my sorrows, my strengths and my doubts, as they arose, without judgment. Yes, I'll celebrate my accomplishments, but not without savoring every step along the way.

How can I be sure that all or any of this has worked? How do I know that this new sense of self-esteem and contentment truly has become an integral part of me? Because for the first time in my life, I stood up for myself and asked for what I wanted. And here's what happened:

For three years on Thursday afternoons, after my *Good Morning America* segment that morning, I have done a local version of

"Deals & Steals" called "Secret Sales" on WABC, the number one–rated local television station in the country. The timing is more relaxed and I often get as much as five minutes of airtime to talk about products, not the two or three minutes on the faster-paced *GMA*. The local spot is also a chance to feature stuff made by smaller businesses that couldn't possibly handle the sales volume generated by vast exposure on national television.

But the best thing about the afternoon segment is the banter with co-anchors Liz Cho and David Novarro and meteorologist Lee Goldberg. Early on in "Secret Sales," I called Lee my "little swirly bun," a name that stuck after I featured a deal on sugary cinnamon buns. Lee and I go back and forth with him playing the straight man to my antics—or vice versa, depending on the week. David is the friendly, consummate pro who goes along with all of it. He's always telling me that his wife, Joanne, loves my stuff. Off-air Liz is as kind to me as she is on TV. She has a big heart and is a beauty. She hosted a cocktail party for me when *The Shift* was published and we share notes about parenting, relationships, and work in email exchanges and over relaxed lunches.

Now my contract is up and my small salary has stayed the same since I was hired—through three contracts. The station bosses never offer a raise, always preempting the potential conversation by citing urgent budget woes, and I never press it. I figure the job adds to my profile, the commute is just a few blocks from my office, and I love the team I work with. Best to let it slide, I think. Looking back, I now I realize that the vulnerable Fat Girl voice inside my head has held me back all this time. I feel so grateful that someone actually likes me enough to put me on TV that I don't dare rock the boat by asking for a penny more. Low self-esteem has cost me in so many ways in my life. And what is particularly unnerving is that my negative self-talk on this singular issue alone runs counter to everything I advise other women to do.

It's time to stand up for myself and ask for more money. It's management's job to keep the purse strings tight and I get that. But buoyed by two years of Shifting and many months of genuine happiness on this new journey, I have a specific number in mind. I want a raise that is realistic and reflects the work I put into the segment, the popularity of "Secret Sales," and the fact that I've never gotten any bump in my pay. I don't have blinders on: I know full well that they might not go for it. Sure, my segment is fun, viewers like it, and the three anchors and I have a blast every Thursday. But it's still just four or five minutes once a week. I'm worth only so much, no matter how much anyone likes me.

I make that point to the lawyer who is representing me but he scoffs at my current salary. He says that I am clearly underpaid and undervalued. Yet when we come up with a number, he also warns me that they could balk and drop me. He agrees with me: just because *we* think I'm worth more doesn't mean *they* will pay me more. I'm okay with that. In fact, I'm comfortable with whatever happens because I'm at a different place now.

I have a sense of self-worth that comes naturally to many women but is new to me. It's not something that I necessarily let other people see, but Peter knows. For so many years he has watched me accept being underpaid for various things because I didn't have the courage or confidence to speak up for myself and ask for more.

I'm not being cavalier: I can ill afford to lose any income, especially with a double dose of college tuition approaching.

But I also have come to believe that money is all about numbers and numbers never end. The comedian Joe E. Lewis once
said, "It doesn't matter whether you are rich or poor—as long
as you've got money." But if money is your sole motivator, you'll
chase happiness forever and you'll never catch it.

Peter and I have talked many times about the irony of me
urging women to speak up for their worth and holding to their
"walk-away" number when I, personally, settle for much less.
Even if they dump me, I decide going in, I will still feel good about
myself. I am sure about that because over the recent months I
have gained a new confidence in myself. It's a feeling I have that
if one thing doesn't work out, something else will. I have come
to be less afraid of being fired, losing a gig, or failing to nab a
specific project or assignment. I realize there are only so many
hours in the day for me to work, and my work time must be spent
on people and projects that truly value my talent and that I enjoy.

After plenty of back-and-forth, the news director goes from
offering a firm "no raise" to finally budging with a minimal one.
We're far apart, and my lawyer and I reject their offer. I assume
there's still some room to talk since I think my number is reasonable, but there's silence. Days later the news director announces
to her troops that I'm out, which I hear about in phone calls
and texts from stunned friends at the station who say they can't
believe I'm leaving. Just weeks earlier, hugging after a lunch, the
news director told me, "I will never lose one of my people before
I have a direct conversation with them." Obviously that never
happened.

I'm sorry it didn't work out, but I have no regrets. I had a
blast finding good deals for local viewers and working with my
on-air pals Liz, David, and Lee. They are still my friends, and

my former colleagues there joke that the table on the set in the studio overlooking Lincoln Center will always be known as Toryville. They tell me repeatedly that I was a great burst of fun every week and they loved the effortless chemistry between us. That part I miss.

But I also know that the end of this gig is not the end of the world. Knowing full well that I could lose this job, I plotted a Plan B: I have worked to secure new consulting clients—a divorce lawyer and a financial advisor—both of whom want my help ramping up their speaking engagements. Those projects will more than make up for the lost income from local TV. Would I have preferred to keep that fun gig *and* land this additional work? Absolutely, but not at the cost of my self-worth.

I'm not the woman I was twenty-two years ago at NBC News, when I was given thirty minutes to leave 30 Rock and escorted out by security guards. Then I holed myself up in my apartment for weeks with the blinds drawn, humiliated that I had been shown the door. I didn't answer calls from friends and I had no interest in meeting new people who inevitably would ask, "Where do you work? What do you do?" Now, when viewers ask me on Facebook what happened to "Secret Sales," instead of ignoring the question, I tell them straight up: "Sorry, it's over. The boss killed it!" No bitterness or anger. It is what it is. I thank them for being loyal watchers.

My mood is also in stark contrast to how I felt after I lost the other potential TV deal. Back then I thought my world would collapse. It didn't, of course, but I still felt I had somehow caused the deal to fall through because I was a mess and didn't have my act together. I've emerged a stronger woman from two career losses in one year and a sudden personal loss the year before. I now have an arsenal of tools I carry to protect me going forward. The news director at WABC tells her staff, but not me, that I am welcome back anytime, if they can make it work. Translation: if I agree to their terms.

She controls the checkbook and I respect that. But I own my confidence, and I respect that much more. Maybe one day we'll find a middle ground.

Days later I find a little charm box on my bed after I get out of the shower. Inside is a diamond double angel-wing necklace and a note that reads:

Dear Mom,
You're the best angel for tons of people and you should know that we love and appreciate you so much and we'll always be your angels.

Love, Emma and Jake

It's now been three years since The Chat, my "lose weight or else" discussion with Barbara Fedida. I've continued to meditate, I sleep better at night, and I'm more focused at work. I'm less anxious these days and not as likely to lose my temper out of frustration. It may sound corny, but after I meditate I encourage myself to think about one new thing that I'm grateful for since the last time I meditated. It's a great way to start and end a day. It doesn't prevent problems from arising, but it keeps things in perspective and stops me from spinning out of control. I've come to believe that when our troubles occupy our mind, they can crush our spirit and suppress our joy. When doom and gloom overtake our thoughts, it's because we refuse to focus on anything else. Instead of letting negative thoughts, roadblocks, and challenges cloud my thinking, I deliberately *choose* to focus on what I'm grateful for. When I do that, invariably I handle problems better. Besides, nothing positive ever comes from panic: worrying solves nothing.

I know now that my *if only* mindset was a crutch. When I made my first Shift, women told me we were sisters from another mother. Perhaps I will now discover new would-be siblings who have been carrying around an *if only* mindset and are ready to let it go. I'm here for them—and you.

After listening to me share stories about my kids for years, my friend Anna Robertson, a new mom, emails me to say, "May we all aspire to have kids who love and appreciate us as much as yours do for you!" My empty-nest worries are over, replaced by the confidence that I'm sending two incredible people into the world—both of whom can and will always come home. Jake has shown me that obstacles are often only in our minds. He has taught himself to swing a golf club in his bedroom after school, via YouTube videos. For a city kid, golf courses are hard to get to, so his carpet, or what's left of it in the spot he's designated as his tee, replaced the putting green. He practices every day: only then can he see change and know what to work on to improve. Emma makes money the old-fashioned way: she earns it. As for Peter, my moon and stars, my everything: if we had to trade it all in for cardboard end tables in our first small apartment again, I'd be happy with him until the end of time. A great marriage is much more than making money, and what he gives me and us as a couple and a family is worth more than any paycheck. As we get closer to an empty nest, I couldn't imagine a better partner to have by my side to navigate this next phase of life.

Whether you're Shifting your weight or Shifting your head

and your heart, I hope that reading about my journey helps you. It took me losing seventy pounds and a series of life crises to tap into the calm, peace, and power that I never knew I had but were inside of me all along. Whatever you dream of doing in coming days, weeks, and months, I hope you nail it. Don't wait until you're at your perfect weight, find the perfect mate, or have that perfect job to start being good to yourself. "Happy is the new black," as one of my favorite T-shirts reads. Your best life starts now, not five or ten pounds from now. Make today Day One by closing this book and thinking not just about what you want to get but also about what you want to give. I've found deep satisfaction in a balance of both.

We all need a portable sense of self-esteem, the confidence to know that no matter what happens to us or around us, we'll be okay. Whether we're facing divorce, an empty nest, job loss, or the death of someone we love, we know we have all we need to support ourselves. I know I am loved: I have a strong family and friendships to prove it. I have learned to relax my mind with acupuncture, meditation, and exercise. I know that I have value because I find joy in giving. There will always be challenges, things that I can't control. But I've learned that I *can* control how I react to those challenges, and if I focus, I can do pretty much anything I set my mind and heart on. I know I have the tools that allow me to refill my well, chart a new course for myself, and try, try again. I'm good with that.

Nobody's coming to rescue us. It's up to each of us to make our dreams happen. You have exactly what it takes to do just that.

Five Steps of Shifting

When I decided to write *Shift for Good*, I didn't want it to be a step-by-step self-help book: I'm not a teacher and I don't have all the answers. Just as *The Shift* is not a diet book, *Shift for Good* is not meant to be the definitive guide to inner peace.

I chose instead to share the journey of what happened to me during a tumultuous year after I had finally lost a lot of weight. Much of what happened came as a shock and surprise to me. I had to act—and that's what I did.

I knew going into this book that I'd have to come clean about aspects of my life that are embarrassing to me, just as writing about my lifetime battle with obesity had been. But I felt that if I could help other women who face challenges similar to mine, it'd be worth it once again. I'm glad I did, and if you've read this far, I held your interest. Thank you.

Looking back at my journey, five specific steps that helped me make my original Shift physically also helped me Shift emotionally. When I lost all that weight, I realized that what I put in my head was far more powerful than what I put in my mouth. This time, I learned that what I fill my head with—the messages I tell myself, and the choices I make—is key to Shifting for Good. I needed to stop thinking of myself as The Fat Girl, and let go of the shame that once defined me. I needed to embrace my strength and own my confidence, regardless of my size and independent of my career prospects. I also realized that I had spent so much time focusing on my weight and my career that I never stopped to think about how to manage my life in ways that would bring lasting contentment—beyond the scale or a paycheck.

By asking and answering these five questions with an honesty that comes from deep within, I think that almost anyone can make a significant change in her life, as I did in mine. If you've read *The Shift*, you'll probably recognize these steps. They helped me jump-start my weight loss Shift, and I've adapted them for my inner quest. You can, too.

STEP ONE: HOW FED UP ARE YOU, REALLY?

In other words, are you finally sick of the way things are now? When I made my first Shift, I was. For the first time in my life, I was sick of avoiding my doctor, being a bad role model for Emma, hating how I looked, and being frustrated that none of my clothes fit. The pain of the present outweighed the pain of change. Change is hard, but for me being overweight was harder. When you're at a point where the pain of the present outweighs the pain and sacrifice that change demands, you're ready to Shift.

This time around, I was fed up with worrying about things I couldn't control, such as a lost TV opportunity, age, illness and death, and an empty nest. I realized that panic doesn't solve anything, nor does it improve the outcome. I was coasting and embarrassed by how that impacted my business, and by extension my family. I cringed at my behavior: from ditching work to snapping at Peter. In order to change for good, ask yourself: How fed up are you?

STEP TWO: WHAT ARE YOU WILLING TO GIVE UP?

Big change requires big sacrifice. No way around it. Dropping sixty-two pounds that first year meant giving up many things I once enjoyed a lot. It wasn't so much the food that did me in; it was my *attitude*. Cheat days and a variety of excuses had to go. Yet many people who want to lose weight or make other big life changes resist making sacrifices. They put up roadblocks that handicap any chance of success before they even start. They refuse to give up a nightly glass of wine, a cigarette after a stressful day, or a weekly pasta dinner. They promise to stick to a plan that they've outlined for themselves—and then cheat at every turn. If you want to Shift for Good, *nothing* can be more important than tackling your goal. You must be willing to give up things that are near and dear to you—including certain behaviors—if you want to succeed. You must be ready to commit fully; be willing to accept the Shift as an all-or-nothing deal, as hard as it sounds. And it *is* hard, but it gets easier to live with over time.

This time, I had to banish the *"if only"* mentality that I'd clung to forever, like a kid giving up a favorite rag doll or blanket. I had to dump my dangerous sense of entitlement and chart a new course. If I was going to succeed, I had to make it happen myself. I had to accept that the world doesn't owe me anything and that life comes with a series of ongoing challenges from the day we're born to the day we die. The grass may seem greener on the other side, but it isn't always. Better to focus on perfecting your own lawn than envying someone else's. Besides, life is beautiful no matter what your lawn looks like.

STEP THREE: WHAT'S YOUR PLAN?

There's no winging it if you're serious about making a significant life change. You need to establish clear, concise rules in order to eliminate ambiguity. Make a simple plan for how you're going to tackle your issue. For me, cutting carbs was the right method to lose weight because I knew from Day One what I could and couldn't eat. That made it very straightforward for me, with no gray areas. I stuck with my plan and it paid off because I knew my parameters: eat less, choose better, move more.

This time, I also created a three-pronged plan for myself. I decided to (1) care for my head and my heart as diligently as I had cared for my body; (2) value my time and talent more, and focus on things that matter in my business and ignore things that don't; and (3) give back regularly, not just seasonally, and revel in the joy of helping people and causes I care about.

STEP FOUR: WHAT'S YOUR DAILY ACCOUNTABILITY?

It's easy to slip up when nobody's looking. It's also possible to fool yourself into thinking that you're on track when you're not. When I was losing weight, daily weigh-ins became my reality check. They still are. A watchful and loving family, changes in clothing size, feedback from colleagues, and photos were good secondary sources of accountability.

This time, those measures of accountability seem more elusive, but they exist. Take a moment to review each day to see which emotions and attitudes reigned: calm or panic, happy or angry, joyful or joyless? If you consistently practice the action steps you outline in your plan, odds are you'll see and feel results. Progress begets progress, which makes daily accountability important.

STEP FIVE: HOW WILL YOU DEVELOP PATIENCE AND CELEBRATE YOUR VICTORIES?

Until I made the Shift, I wasn't nearly patient or persistent enough to make a dent in my weight. I always gave up too soon. I succeeded only when I decided to view my Shift not as a diet but as a journey toward wholeness that would take time. To stay motivated, I began to celebrate teeny victories—often with non-edible rewards so I wouldn't derail my success. I learned that change rarely happens in a flash or even on a timetable.

This time was no different. It's hard to go from panic to perfect overnight, no matter how much we want it to work that way. My greatest victories now include feeling a level of contentment that I didn't even know existed. I'm learning to be more patient and generous with myself—and others—and I try to treat myself as if I were my own best friend. There's no end date on my plan. I intend to use all of my tools—from meditation to giving back—to move from "fed up" to "fabulous," and I'm in it for the long haul. I'm betting that the rewards from all of it will increase over time.

Six Parts Make a Whole

I've spent many months trying all the stuff I've talked about in this book, implementing new thoughts and daily routines. There's so much debate about whether or not women can have it all—a happy family and a great career—to create a fulfilling life for themselves. As my kids are poised to graduate from high school, I can reflect on the last eighteen years and say with certainty that I was blessed to have had both. But I've now changed my definition of "having it all" to focus not just on two areas, but on six. Paying attention to all of them helps me feel content and whole.

1. **Love and relationships:** I want to love and be loved and I'm willing to put in the effort to make that happen, especially since I know that maintaining strong relationships takes work.

2. **Healthy mind and body:** I want to treat my body with the love and respect it deserves, and I want to create a calm mind that focuses more on the present moment and less on the past and future—neither of which I can control.

3. **Satisfying work and wealth:** This is not about being rich or amassing hordes of cash. I spend so much time working that

I want my work to matter to me and to the people I serve. I crave peace of mind around financial security and I will never lose sight of money matters.

4. **Impact through giving:** Lending my time and talent to people in need fills my head and heart with happiness and joy. There's no such thing as too much of this, and I want to participate as fully as I can and as often as I'm able.

5. **Calm environment:** While outside chaos can't always be contained, I recognize that I have full control over my home and work surroundings. I choose to make both havens of harmony, not disruption.

6. **Curiosity in action:** This is the antidote to boredom. I want to wake up curious every single day. I want that curiosity to lead me to interesting places, near and far, and to fuel my desire to do great things that will make a difference in the world.

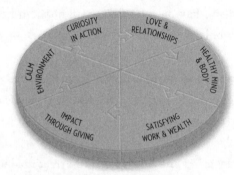

100 Things I Crave

Melody Biringer, founder of Seattle's Urban Campfire, the event where Emma dared me to be oh-so-bold on stage, believes that women focus on everyone else's needs and desires to the exclusion of their own. She says we should reflect not just on our big bucket list but also on the small stuff that makes us happy. She encourages women to create a list of the things they crave because it forces them to put time and thought into moments that inspire joy inside and out. This exercise allows you to reflect on what turns you on. Below is my list of 100 things that I enjoy because they always make me smile. It has become one of my favorite Pinterest boards and I encourage you to create one for yourself. Take some time to design your own list of things that help you to be good to yourself—and share it with me using #ShiftforGood.

1. Neon "don't mess with me" Nikes
2. Mr. Bubble bubble baths
3. Cuticle oil to make manicures look like new
4. Impromptu dance parties alone at home
5. Grapefruit-scented body scrub
6. Watching *Legally Blonde*

7. Adding a mini gold star to one nail
8. Reading *Oprah* magazine
9. Pistachios
10. Black long-lash drugstore mascara
11. Putting my hair up after a long day
12. Lighting scented candles
13. Wearing my GOAL DIGGER T-shirt
14. Taking long walks in Central Park
15. Spending an afternoon at the Museum of Natural History
16. Sipping cappuccino with a friend
17. Traveling
18. Gazing at the ocean
19. Walking on the beach
20. Twenty-minute meditations
21. Custom journals from May Designs
22. Snuggling with Marly
23. Swimming on a blazing hot day
24. Short-interval strength training
25. Getting a good night's sleep
26. Clear lip gloss
27. Stella perfume
28. Mushrooms
29. Acupuncture facial
30. Marathon texting session with a great friend
31. Light pink nail polish
32. Fresh flowers
33. Fluffy pillows
34. Experimenting with low-carb recipes
35. Plush towels

36. Long, hot showers
37. Blaring pop songs and singing along
38. At-home peel-off face masks
39. Homemade guacamole
40. Blow-outs for straight hair
41. Art supplies
42. Treadmill desk
43. Self-tanner
44. Hair-thickening mousse
45. Playing Scrabble
46. Grapefruit slices
47. Creating photo albums
48. Posting positive quotes
49. Road trips
50. Family dinners
51. Melted Brie and celery
52. Broadway musicals
53. Metallic Sharpies
54. Zucchini "noodles" as a pasta substitute
55. Exploring on Instagram
56. Flea markets and antiques shows
57. Snapping selfies with my kids
58. Reading the *New York Post*
59. Citrus-scented hand cream
60. Pedicures
61. Cozy sweatpants
62. Handwritten notes
63. Balloons
64. Holiday celebrations with family and friends

65. Mint dental floss

66. Light jogs in the park

67. Watching awards shows

68. Three-generation lunches with my mom and Emma

69. Designing jewelry

70. Fund-raising

71. Scratch-off lottery tickets

72. Dreaming about fantasy vacations

73. Starbucks iced coffee with extra ice

74. Water infused with lemon

75. Dentyne Fire sugar-free gum

76. Watching Beyoncé or Katy Perry perform

77. Flipping through photo albums

78. Walking around the Metropolitan Museum of Art

79. Searching for new products for my segments

80. Amelia Rose earrings

81. Sour pickles

82. Hail Merry chocolate chip macaroons

83. Rosemary and garlic roasted chicken

84. Browsing *InStyle* magazine

85. *Good Morning America* summer concerts in Central Park

86. Fresh popcorn

87. Rose-scented face cream

88. Roaming the aisles in Target

89. Roasted and shelled pistachios

90. Monograms

91. Creating decoupage plates

92. Giving unexpected gifts to girlfriends

93. Watching TV in a crowded bed with my family

94. Occasional headstands

95. Strolling along the Hudson River
96. Fishing with Jake
97. Helping Emma with her business
98. Playing dress-up with our tiaras
99. Fireworks
100. Jawbone activity tracker

Acknowledgments

It takes a village to turn my experiences into a book and I'm grateful to everyone on my side, starting with the exceptional team at Hachette Books: publisher Mauro DiPreta, executive editor Stacy Creamer, executive director of publicity Michelle Aielli, marketing director Betsy Hulsebosch, art director Christopher Lin, production editor Melanie Gold, copyeditor Katherine Ness, and editorial assistant Lauren Hummel. The sales team always delivers and I'm especially thankful for Chris Murphy, Dave Epstein, Karen Torres, and Mike Heuer. Linda Sparrowe, Dana Lynch, and Jodi Goldman offered candid feedback and skillful editing. Heidi Krupp is my literary warrior. To my ABC News and *Good Morning America* family: it's an honor to work among the smartest, most dedicated people anywhere. Photographers Ida Astute and Heidi Gutman at ABC are picture-perfect in my book. I'm indebted to Barbara Fedida at ABC News, who inspired the first Shift and has kept me moving in the right direction ever since. To Gianna Fata, my valued colleague who makes everything work week after week, my gratitude and friendship. Peter, Emma, Jake, and Nick: I love and treasure you. And to every person who has read my books, watched me on TV, attended one of my events, or connected me with on social media: I appreciate your trust in me and I value your interest in what I do. Austin Gasparini—you can now cross off your bucket list goal of seeing your name in print.

CONNECT WITH ME

I would love to hear from you. Share your Shift with me anytime at ToryJohnson.com or socially at Facebook.com/Tory or @ToryJohnson on Twitter, Instagram, and Periscope.

Honest, thoughtful, and often hilarious…
I couldn't put this book down.

—*Gretchen Rubin, bestselling author of*
The Happiness Project

LEARN HOW THE SHIFT BEGAN.

Read Tory Johnson's #1
New York Times best seller
The Shift today.

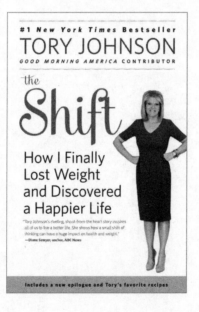

Also Available as an eBook and from Hachette Audio

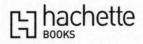